Synthesis Lectures on Threatcasting

Series Editors

Brian David Johnson, Arizona State University, Tempe, USA

Natalie Vanatta, United States Military Academy, West Point, USA

This series publishes short books that explore the analytical method of threatcasting, which draws on a wide range of fields to develop techniques for recognizing future threats, designing potential futures, and exposing events that could indicate the progression toward an increasingly possible threat landscape. Books in this series will cover all aspects of the threatcasting methodology for researchers and practitioners. The series will promote new dialogues across a variety of communities and keep up to date with novel developments in the area.

Melissa Smallwood

The Future of Long COVID

A Threatcasting Approach

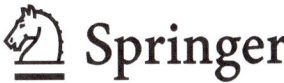

Springer

Melissa Smallwood
School for the Future of Innovation in Society
Arizona State University
Phoenix, AZ, USA

ISSN 2771-1560   ISSN 2771-1579   (electronic)
Synthesis Lectures on Threatcasting
ISBN 978-3-031-40473-3   ISBN 978-3-031-40474-0   (eBook)
https://doi.org/10.1007/978-3-031-40474-0

This Springer imprint is published by the registered company Springer Nature Switzerland AG
The registered company address is: Gewerbestrasse 11, 6330 Cham, Switzerland

Contents

Introduction

The COVID-19 pandemic is an ongoing catastrophe that has disrupted the global economy, worsened existing social tensions and inequalities, and caused over 6.4 million deaths globally (World Health Organization [WHO] 2021). From the start of the pandemic in March 2020, media attention and political response to the crisis have focused largely on its most dramatic and disruptive short-term aspects. However, little attention has been paid to the fact that the COVID-19 pandemic is one of the largest mass-disabling events of the modern era.

An estimated 20–30% of people infected with this highly contagious illness experience long-term post-infectious symptoms and an increased risk of serious medical complications—a collection of illnesses that have come to be known as "Long COVID" or "Post-Acute Sequelae of COVID-19" (PASC). Long COVID became a recognized medical phenomenon due to the advocacy of large online networks formed by COVID survivors who experienced lingering illness and disability months after their initial infections in 2020.

These patient advocates, who refer to themselves as "Long Haulers," lobbied medical providers, government agencies, and media outlets to acknowledge the reality and seriousness of their condition. As of 2022, three years into the pandemic, Long COVID continues to challenge the dominant narrative that "mild cases" of COVID-19 (those not resulting in hospitalization or death) do not pose any significant long-term risks.

The long-term impact of Long COVID and the COVID-19 pandemic as a whole is unknown, but each new infection adds to the magnitude of the pandemic's eventual impact. The Centers for Disease Control and Prevention (CDC) estimates that more than 24 million Americans, or 7.5% of the population, may be experiencing Long COVID as of

M. Smallwood, *The Future of Long COVID*, Synthesis Lectures on Threatcasting, https://doi.org/10.1007/978-3-031-40474-0_1

summer 2022 (Center for Disease Control and Prevention 2022). Other surveys accounting for the large number of unreported COVID cases estimate that the true burden of post-COVID illness may be even higher than this staggering figure.

These newly acquired disabilities impact not only the individuals experiencing them, but also their families, communities, businesses, and societal-level institutions. The ripple effects of population-level Long COVID are concerning, given that social safety net systems meant to address them are underfunded, inefficient, and politicized. As long-haulers reckon with an uncertain future, many worry that the effects of poor policy choices may be as devastating to their lives as the illness itself.

This book uses Threatcasting—a participatory scenario-planning methodology that models threats and futures in a complex and uncertain environment (Johnson et al. 2021)—to study the long-term effects of Long COVID on large societal systems and institutions and identify specific actions that can be taken to mitigate these effects. Including COVID long-haulers as scenario-planning participants and incorporating their lived experience as a form of expertise—alongside more conventional subject matter experts from fields such as public health, epidemiology, information science, workforce development, and strategic planning—is crucial to this study.

A total of 24 study participants were split into groups and asked to collectively develop scenarios focusing on a specific person experiencing a specific threat related to Long COVID in the year 2031—ten years into the future. The groups then linked the scenarios back to present-day reality and produced indicators/actions that could be used to warn, prevent, mitigate, or help recover from the future threat. This exercise helps in identifying and assessing long-term challenges that Long COVID—as a form of widespread disability on a population level—presents to communities, systems, and institutions within the United States (US).

This book is a first step in moving the conversation on Long COVID beyond that of an individualized medical problem and toward assessing the collective impact of this new condition.

1.1   How to Use This Book

The Threatcasting project that forms the basis of this book was conducted for the Master of Science and Technology Policy program at Arizona State University. In some ways, it is an attempt to glimpse into the future during a time of great uncertainty. In other ways, the project is a time capsule—a snapshot into a specific part of the pandemic that can only do so much to predict the specific and bizarre ways that things have fallen apart since then. Both are important.

My research for this book and the Threatcasting project has been deeply influenced by my background in interdisciplinary neuroscience, psychology, and social science, and my work in autism—particularly regarding the scientific and popular media narratives that contributed to stigmatizing attitudes against autistic people and fed into harmful misinformation, such as that of the anti-vaccine movement. Throughout this work, I was interested in the tense relationship between autistic self-advocates and the autism research community, as well as other patient groups whose needs and priorities were unaligned or in conflict with dominant research paradigms. It was here that I first heard about the struggles faced by people with Myalgic Encephalomyelitis/Chronic Fatigue Syndrome (ME/CFS) and other poorly understood chronic illnesses. When these patient groups sounded the alarm early in the COVID-19 pandemic, before the rest of the public understood how bad this outbreak could get, I began thinking about what the consequences of widespread complex disability could be for our society.

The type of threat that Long COVID poses is not something that the average person or average government is equipped to handle. Our brain has evolved to react to immediate threats to one's life or well-being and is ill-equipped to conceive of complex, long-term risks; even if such risks carry the threat of future suffering, death, or societal breakdown. As an example, just ask a climate scientist about how well humanity is dealing with climate change. One of the goals of this book, and the Threatcasting framework that underlies it, is to establish a structure that will better enable people to think about the long-term impacts of Long COVID and other ripple effects of the pandemic, and the ways that these may interact with other issues within society.

Threatcasting, as a framework, is meant to be future-facing with a focus on issues and threats that will play out over the years, and the perspectives offered in this book are intended to encourage thinking about the aftereffects of COVID-19 long after the acute stage of the pandemic has passed. At the same time, as the COVID-19 pandemic continues to evolve and develop chaotically, some of the issues raised in this book provide only a snapshot of a particular time and place—specifically, autumn 2021 in the US, with edits and updates being made in summer 2022. The main developments in the pandemic between these two time periods include:

1. *The rise and rapid spread of the Omicron variants—a family of hyper-contagious and immune-evasive mutants not descended from previous variants*. Some of the challenges introduced by this variant were anticipated in the Threatcasting project even though the variant did not exist at the time. The challenges range from immune-evasive variants that reduce vaccine efficacy to reinfections, co-circulation of multiple variants, the dismantling of the testing and surveillance apparatus, widespread infection of children and young adults, and normalization and complacency toward the virus.

2. *Inadequate research on Long COVID*. Although the Threatcasting project has called for research into Long COVID multiple times, progress remains slow and has yet to result in FDA-approved treatments and diagnostics. However, significant headway has been made in identifying potential biomarkers and treatment targets. This research has been a global effort and some projects have relied on private actors and crowdfunded campaigns for funding instead of the traditional scientific funding apparatus.

3. ***Slow legislative action on Long COVID***. More congressional legislation on Long COVID has been introduced on top of the two bills that existed in Autumn 2021, although all these bills are yet to be passed. Senator Tim Kaine (D) was the first member of Congress to publicly admit experiencing Long COVID symptoms in March 2022 and has used his experiences to push for more action on Long COVID in the Senate.

This book is meant to start a conversation about Long COVID beyond the current perspective as a medical problem that atomized individuals must cope with on their own. To comprehend and prepare for the impact that a health crisis of this scale may have on our society, we must shift our thinking beyond the short-term crises created by the pandemic and separate the systemic impacts of widespread chronic illness from those of widespread acute illness. This includes looking at Long COVID from multiple angles—not just a medical lens—and bringing together perspectives from different subject matter experts to explore how the impacts of this illness intersect with other societal issues. Long COVID and its impacts on individuals and communities need to be thought of as a policy issue in addition to a medical one. The goal of this book is to help policymakers, researchers, medical professionals, patient advocates, and anyone else who wants to help move toward a solution for Long COVID expand and frame their thinking on this issue.

This book is also intended to document and preserve perspectives from earlier on in the pandemic. Most of the documentation about COVID-19 and Long COVID—such as news stories, statistics, conversations within patient groups, or fears being shared by people across the world—took place online. It can be difficult to find specific information from the early days of the pandemic. Despite only happening two years ago, much of the information generated about the pandemic existed within an ecosystem of dynamically-updated news sites and social media platforms—leaving questions about what happened in 2020 and 2021 to embodied knowledge and fallible memory. At the same time, the pandemic and its mitigations—such as masking, testing, and even booster vaccinations—are disappearing rapidly from public life, and a concerted effort to rewrite the narrative around COVID-19 is in full swing. The magnitude of Long COVID has been scarcely acknowledged by government agencies and major media outlets. However, in the same breath, these authorities proclaim that the pandemic is over and call to return to the status quo at all costs. This rewriting of history is neither new nor unique—a similar social death occurred with the 1918 influenza pandemic, the deadliest disease event of the twentieth century. Although this book and the project that spawned it are focused on the future, it also provides an important glimpse into the past—when the pandemic was still at the top of peoples' minds.

References

Center for Disease Control and Prevention (CDC) (2022) Nearly one in five American adults who have had COVID-19 still have long COVID. https://www.cdc.gov/nchs/pressroom/nchs_press_releases/2022/20220622.htm. Accessed 10 Sept 2022

Johnson BD, Vanatta N, Coon C (2021) Threatcasting: Synthesis lectures on threatcasting. Morgan & Claypool, San Rafael

World Health Organization (WHO) (2021). WHO Coronavirus (COVID-19) Dashboard. https://covid19.who.int. Accessed 20 June 2022

What Is Long Covid?

2

Long COVID, also known as Post-Acute Sequelae of COVID-19 (PASC),[1] is a post-infectious condition characterized by a range of persistent symptoms and a "lack of return to a usual state of health" following a COVID-19 infection (CDC 2021). The symptoms and severity of Long COVID can vary widely between individuals, making it difficult to establish diagnostic criteria that are sufficiently inclusive. Adding to this challenge is the fact that Long COVID and other medical complications, such as organ damage, can emerge in a substantial minority of people who had mild or even asymptomatic cases of COVID-19. Due to substantial undertesting of COVID cases throughout the pandemic, the number of people who may ultimately be affected by post-COVID medical complications is not known.

2.1   Symptoms

Post-COVID medical complications or sequelae can vary widely in the symptoms experienced, the organ systems impacted, and the severity of the illness. Some of the commonly reported symptoms in post-COVID patients more than six months after initial infection, as reported by the CDC and WHO (Chung et al. 2021), include the following:

---

[1] I will be referring to this condition as "Long COVID" for the remainder of this book, because this is the preferred terminology of the long-hauler patient advocates who participated in this project, as well as the most widely known name for the condition. "PASC" is used more frequently within medical and scientific circles.

© The Author(s), under exclusive license to Springer Nature Switzerland AG 2024   7
M. Smallwood, *The Future of Long COVID*, Synthesis Lectures on Threatcasting,
https://doi.org/10.1007/978-3-031-40474-0_2

- Shortness of breath
- Fatigue
- Exercise intolerance
- Cognitive dysfunction ("Brain fog")
- Cough
- Chest or stomach pain
- Headache
- Heart palpitations

- Dysautonomia/postural orthostatic tachycardia syndrome (POTS)
- Joint or muscle pain
- Neuropathy
- Sleep disturbances
- Rash
- Loss of taste or smell

Approximately one-third of post-COVID patients in existing studies report at least one lingering symptom six months after their initial infection. A study examining the health records of over 273,000 post-COVID patients found that 57% of patients reported at least one of nine major symptoms associated with Long COVID in the six-month period following their recovery from acute infection. Within this sample, 36% of post-COVID patients reported at least one lingering symptom more than three months after infection, with 7.94% of the patients reporting difficulty breathing, 5.87% experiencing fatigue, and 15.49% reporting anxiety or depression six months after infection (Taquet et al. 2021). Another study of over 70,000 post-COVID patients conducted using data from the Veterans Health Administration (VHA) found elevated disease burden across 12 diagnosis categories—especially for respiratory, cardiac, circulatory, nervous, and metabolic disorders—as well as an increase in general ill-health (Al-Aly et al. 2021). These disease symptoms were reinforced by numerous laboratory abnormalities.

In addition to studies that examine the prevalence of common post-COVID symptoms in the general post-COVID population, surveys conducted by long-hauler patient groups have found a broad and heterogeneous range of symptoms. One of the largest patient-led studies, which included over 3,000 people linked to online long-hauler support groups, identified 205 symptoms across ten affected organ systems (Davis et al. 2021). Patient-led research conducted within long-hauler support networks has uncovered substantial levels of newly acquired disability within this population. People with no preexisting health conditions before infection have reported new diagnoses across more than ten organ systems.

This disease burden has occurred alongside a drastic decline in health and quality of life (self-reported). Some of the most debilitating symptoms reported by long-haulers include severe energy limitations that prevent them from working or completing routine, everyday activities without inducing exhaustion and cognitive dysfunction that is commonly known as "brain fog." Examples of cognitive errors described by members of a Long COVID Patient Group (2022) include the following:

I was driving home from work and lost track of where I was. I couldn't remember what exit I needed to take to get home. I had to call my spouse and have him guide me home by phone. I have lived in my home for 21 years.

A few months ago, I wanted to call one of my best friends that I've talked to every day for the last two years. Couldn't remember her name. I had to scroll through all of my recent conversations and say their names out loud until I realized which one was her and then, I broke down and cried. That is not normal.

When I would drive, I couldn't recognize lights changing or notice stop signs.

There have been occasions where I am looking at my 7-year-old daughter and I can't remember her name.

For many with Long COVID, the distress experienced from symptoms is compounded by a loss of autonomy, identity, and social role. The transition—from one's life before COVID infection to after—can be extremely sudden, occurring in a matter of weeks or months, and the severity of the disability that can occur is jarring, especially in cases with a mild acute infection.

Many people experiencing Long COVID symptoms are in the younger to middle age group, with prior good health and little experience with disability. Other long-haulers are people with previously controlled medical conditions that have been exacerbated or have begun acting unpredictably after a COVID infection. In either case, people with Long COVID must navigate becoming unexpectedly ill with little medical or social support and no clear solutions.

Research into why Long COVID causes such a wide and heterogenous range of symptoms is ongoing. Long COVID's effects across organ systems resemble the symptom variations seen in acute COVID infection. While acute COVID-19 is often characterized as a respiratory illness, it can target a range of organ systems, including the cardiac, circulatory, gastrointestinal, nervous, and renal systems. The SARS-COV-2 virus can affect many different parts of our body as it binds itself to the body's ACE2 receptor, which is involved in regulating inflammation in most of the body's organ systems (Scialo et al. 2020; Baig et al. 2020). Research on the biological underpinnings of Long COVID, which has been released since the completion of the Threatcasting pilot project, has found numerous potential explanations for Long COVID's systemic effects. These findings include the following:

1. Abnormal clotting pathology and vascular inflammation causing microscopic blood clots and hypoxia (Pretorius et al. 2021);
2. Viral persistence in organ systems such as the gastrointestinal tract (Wang et al. 2020);
3. Autoantibodies indicating an ongoing autoimmune response (Seeßle et al. 2021);

4. Multiple pathways for neurological symptoms including direct infection of the nervous system through the olfactory nerve (Bougakov et al. 2021);
5. Dysfunction and exhaustion of CD4+ and CD8+ T-cells (Wiech et al. 2022; Patterson et al. 2021); and
6. Reactivation of dormant viral infections such as Epstein-Barr Virus (EBV) (Gold et al. 2021).

These findings are not mutually exclusive, and multiple biological abnormalities could be the source of Long COVID's variable symptoms.

2.2   Prevalence

Estimates of the percentage of COVID survivors who go on to develop Long COVID vary but tend to average between 10 and 30% of patients (CDC 2022), with complication rates being higher for people infected early in the pandemic, and reduced—but not eliminated—for people infected post-vaccination (Thaweethai et al. 2023). The development of Long COVID symptoms is not contingent on the severity of the initial infection, although people with severe illness are at greater risk of developing long-term complications. Much of the initial research on Long COVID specifically focused on lingering symptoms experienced by patients who had been hospitalized for COVID infection—a group that makes up approximately 14% of total COVID cases (CDC 2021).

Hospitalization due to COVID-19 infection is associated with worse health outcomes and higher rates of readmission, disability, and death (Ayoubkhani et al. 2021; PHOSP-COVID Collaborative Group et al. 2021). This correlation can be attributed to both a more severe initial infection and the risks added due to the hospitalization process. However, many Long COVID cases occur among people with initially mild or even asymptomatic infection. A study exploring the risk factors associated with developing Long COVID found that 32% of non-hospitalized long-haulers reported an asymptomatic initial COVID infection (Huang et al. 2022). Given that 80% of symptomatic COVID cases are considered "mild," much of the total disease burden of Long COVID is occurring in populations that have not been heavily studied and surveilled throughout the pandemic.

The relatively high prevalence of post-infectious symptoms in COVID-19 survivors becomes an alarming statistic when the SARS-COV-2 virus's high rate of transmissibility and rapid spread around the world is considered. In November 2021, over 47 million cases of COVID-19 had been reported in the US, and over 250 million cases worldwide (Allen et al. 2021; WHO 2021). This number jumped after the first Omicron surge to 75 million cases in the US by February 2022 and is at over 93 million cases (600 million globally) as of August 2022. However, these numbers are believed to drastically underestimate the true toll of COVID-19 due to persistent underreporting of COVID cases throughout the pandemic. The underreporting of COVID cases is attributable to multiple causes, some of which are due to policy choices and supply chain issues, while others are related to characteristics of the disease itself.

Approximately 35% of COVID cases are asymptomatic and most patients experience only mild symptoms and recover at home (Sah et al. 2021). Because of the overloading of healthcare systems and the deprioritization of medical interventions for non-severe COVID cases, many people with mild COVID infections may not seek out healthcare or get tested for the disease, instead opting to let the illness pass on its own (Rahmandad et al. 2021). In the early months of the pandemic, the CDC's restrictions on the limited supply of COVID tests for only symptomatic patients meant that many asymptomatic infected people were unable to get tested—a policy that contributed heavily to the pandemic's initial explosion within the US (Shear et al. 2021). Throughout the pandemic, public health officials have been aware of the undertesting and underreporting of COVID cases, particularly among those with asymptomatic infection, but have not been able to act on it.

In the absence of randomized population-level testing, two measures can indirectly be used to assess the prevalence of COVID infection—the positivity rate, and the seroprevalence rate. The positivity rate refers to the percentage of COVID tests within an area that return a positive result, and is used to infer the true prevalence of COVID within a particular area. In standard epidemiological practice, a positivity rate above 5% is considered a threshold that indicates unchecked community transmission and insufficient testing to detect all cases (Dowdy and D'Souza 2020).

In communities where positivity rates of an infectious disease exceed 5%, public health officials typically recommend forms of mitigation such as mask-wearing, school closures, or restrictions on large gatherings. In the US, the COVID positivity rate was far more than the 5% threshold at multiple points in the pandemic—during the winter 2020 peak, nearly every state in the nation experienced unchecked community transmission, with some heavily impacted states reporting positivity rates over 25%. In the winter of 2021, during the first Omicron surge, positivity and case rates obliterated the previous records set in the winter of 2020. As newer Omicron variants have continued to evolve and circulate throughout 2022 and 2023, the average positivity rate in most states has plateaued to around 8–10%—lower than the most dramatic surges, but still well above the previously-recommended 5% threshold.

A second measure that can be used to assess the rate of past COVID-19 infection is the seroprevalence rate. Seroprevalence testing looks for the presence of COVID-19 antibodies in blood samples taken from a segment of the population within a region. Seroprevalence testing in most surveys has focused on antibodies that are produced due to natural infection, which exhibit distinct features from antibodies produced as a result of vaccination. This method of testing provides a more representative sample of the population than testing for active COVID-19 infection since it takes a random sample of the population instead of self-selecting for people with active symptoms or known exposure.

Seroprevalence also provides a picture of COVID infection rates over time, instead of one particular instance. In July 2021, when the Threatcasting pilot project was conducted, the CDC's seroprevalence data estimated that 20% of the sampled US population had been infected with COVID-19. This percentage created an estimate of 66.5 million COVID infections—almost twice the rate of the reported 35 million infections at the end of July 2021. By January 2022, seroprevalence-based models estimated that 106 million Americans—or one in three—had been infected with COVID-19 (Dunne et al. 2022) and studies from the spring of 2022 estimate that nearly 60% of Americans have been infected with the virus.

The CDC ended its community seroprevalence survey in February 2022 due to this data set reaching saturation. With most people in the US having been infected at least once, and many experiencing reinfections from immune-evasive Omicron variants, seroprevalence ceased to be a dynamic and useful metric for measuring the spread of the virus.

As of summer 2022, the CDC estimates that 24 million Americans, or 1 in 13 people, are experiencing long-term medical complications from COVID-19 (CDC 2022). This estimate is based on the number of reported COVID-19 cases in the US and the assumption that 20% of COVID survivors will experience long-term symptoms. Other models, such as those that place the prevalence of Long COVID at 30% or use seroprevalence data to try and account for undetected infections, suggest that this percentage might be higher. Even the most conservative estimates of Long COVID prevalence indicate a substantial increase in long-term disability in the US that existing healthcare and safety net systems are not equipped to handle.

2.3   Notable Comorbidities and Associated Conditions

Long COVID is both a new and old condition. The virus that triggers the illness, SARS-COV-2, is only a few years old and much remains unknown about its long-term health effects. However, many of the symptoms experienced by people with Long COVID overlap with other forms of post-infectious and complex chronic illness that have existed for much longer. Common viral infections like the Epstein-Barr Virus, cytomegalovirus, Lyme disease, and even influenza can cause an out-of-control immune reaction that leads to symptoms such as persistent aches and pains, malaise, fatigue, and exercise intolerance (SMA 2021; Burrell et al. 2017). COVID-19 likely acts as a trigger for these symptoms—except with a much higher attack rate than other common viruses.

Infection-Associated Chronic Illnesses (IACIs)[2] are notoriously difficult to diagnose and treat effectively for multiple reasons. Many of the symptoms associated with post-infectious illness are general symptoms that can potentially be caused by a range of medical conditions. There are no definitive diagnostic tests for many types of post-infectious illness, so the diagnosis requires a process of elimination to rule out other explanations. Additionally, accurate diagnosis requires confirmation of previous viral illness, and awareness on the part of the patient or the practitioner that post-infectious illness exists and is a possible explanation for the symptoms.

Prior to the world-disrupting crisis of the COVID-19 pandemic, most cases of post-viral illness were caused by common viruses from which most patients make a full and uncomplicated recovery. Long-term complications arising from these common infections were seen as a rare occurrence that, in some cases, couldn't be definitively linked to a particular event. Before COVID, many people were simply not aware of post-infectious illness as a possibility, unless someone they knew was disabled by such a condition and could link their disability back to an inciting infection. Due to the difficulties in identifying and diagnosing IACIs, the true prevalence and disease burden of these illnesses is unknown and under-researched. The COVID-19 pandemic has forced the medical and research communities to play catch-up on understanding the causes and treatments for IACIs—a move those members of long-neglected chronic illness communities do not hesitate to point out.

2.3.1 Myalgic Encephalomyelitis (ME/CFS)

ME/CFS is a chronic, multisystemic illness that is characterized by persistent exhaustion, exercise intolerance, cognitive impairment, and an intractable feeling of malaise (NIH 2011; Institute of Medicine 2015). An estimated 40–50% of Long COVID patients meet the diagnostic criteria for ME/CFS (Bonilla et al. 2022; Mancini et al. 2021), leading to an increased focus on ME/CFS as the best available glimpse into what the future might hold for Long COVID patients. The overlap between Long COVID and ME/CFS paints a grim picture due to Long COVID patients inheriting multiple ongoing medical controversies surrounding ME/CFS. These issues include the following:

---

2 "Infection-Associated Chronic Illnesses" (IACIs) is an emerging consensus term for the family of complex/multisystemic chronic illnesses that are triggered by infectious disease. These conditions include Long COVID, ME/CFS, chronic Lyme, multiple sclerosis, and POTS/dysautonomia. The label IACI is being used by the National Academies (NASEM) and other scientific bodies to call for a more comprehensive and unified research agenda on this category of illnesses (NASEM 2023).

1. The persistent lack of research funding, biomarkers, diagnostic tests, and treatments available for ME/CFS;
2. The potential harm caused by exercise-based rehabilitation programs for Long COVID patients with comorbid ME/CFS; and
3. The ongoing struggle of ME/CFS patients, particularly those from marginalized or minority groups, to be taken seriously by the medical establishment.

However, some ME/CFS advocates see a silver lining to the overlap between Long COVID and ME/CFS—in that the research funding and attention being put toward Long COVID may lead to new understandings and treatments for ME/CFS and other neglected post-infectious illnesses.

ME/CFS is considered a severe and debilitating form of chronic illness that negatively impacts all areas of life. The defining symptom of ME/CFS is Post-Exertional Malaise (PEM)—an extreme form of exercise intolerance in which routine daily activities such as cooking a meal, doing laundry, or climbing stairs can lead to exhaustion and a worsening of other ME/CFS symptoms. An estimated 25% of people with ME/CFS are bedbound or housebound by their illness, while others lead more active lives but can suffer from relapses or episodes of severe illness (Pendergrast et al. 2016).

The social and emotional impacts of ME/CFS extend beyond the physiological distress caused by recurrent symptoms—sufferers are often unable to work; face disbelief and denial about their symptoms from friends, family, and medical providers; and can experience a loss of autonomy, identity, and the ability to participate in public life (Asbring 2001; Araja et al. 2021). Research into the quality of life reported by people with ME/CFS has uncovered profound gaps in physical and social functioning when compared to the general population (Eaton-Fitch et al. 2020).

The presence of PEM in the 40–50% of Long COVID patients who meet the criteria for ME/CFS has raised concerns within patient advocate communities due to the emphasis many Long COVID rehabilitation programs place on physical rehabilitation and exercise. The use of Graded Exercise Therapy (GET) as a treatment for ME/CFS is a long-standing medical controversy surrounding this illness (Blease and Geraghty 2018). ME/CFS patients allege that the use of graded exercise is actively harmful to patients with PEM, due to dysfunctional energy metabolism that causes these patients to experience energy crashes, and sometimes, permanent worsening of their illness in response to exercise.

Similarly controversial is the use of Cognitive Behavioral Therapy (CBT) in conjunction with GET. Patients believe this treatment paradigm reinforces the perception that ME/CFS is a psychosomatic disorder, and ignores the serious physiological reality of the disease. Despite the ME/CFS community's opposition to the GET/CBT paradigm, medical guidelines for ME/CFS have only recently begun moving away from these interventions. Many medical practitioners receive little medical education about ME/CFS and other IACIs, and may believe in outdated ideas about these illnesses and their treatments.

These gaps in knowledge continue to influence the current medical response to Long COVID.

People with ME/CFS have a tense and complex relationship with medical providers and the healthcare system. Their debilitating symptoms and complex medical needs place them in frequent contact with the healthcare system, but medical practitioners are often unable or unwilling to adequately address their concerns. Research by the National Institute of Medicine (IOM) estimates that 90% of ME/CFS cases are undiagnosed, with rates of underdiagnosis and unreported cases being especially high in ethnic minority communities (Institute of Medicine 2015; Bayliss et al. 2014). ME/CFS patients, especially women and ethnic minorities, frequently report medical gaslighting and other negative interactions with healthcare providers in which the severity of their symptoms is dismissed or attributed to stigmatized causes such as psychosomatic illness, malingering, or drug-seeking behavior (Guise et al. 2010; Asbring and Narvanen 2003). Even when ME/CFS patients receive a diagnosis, they may still face barriers to adequate care when interacting with multiple specialists or insurance providers.

ME/CFS is a complex, systemic illness that is rarely diagnosed alone. The sections below discuss some of the most common comorbid conditions that are seen among ME/CFS and Long COVID patients. Many of these conditions are frequently triggered by a viral infection, and their rate of co-occurrence raises questions about common underlying pathology and possible genetic risk factors for the development of post-infectious illness.

2.3.2 Dysautonomia and Post Orthostatic Tachycardia Syndrome (POTS)

Dysautonomia, the dysregulation of the autonomic nervous system, is a post-infectious symptom that is very common among Long COVID patients—with two-thirds of one study of over 2,000 patients exhibiting moderate to severe autonomic dysfunction (Larsen et al. 2022). The autonomic nervous system is the part of the nervous system that controls involuntary bodily functions, and dysregulation of this system can cause debilitating symptoms across organ systems. Common dysautonomia symptoms include heart palpitations, spikes in heart rate or blood pressure, dizziness, trouble standing, excessive sweating and temperature dysregulation, gastrointestinal distress, headaches, and fainting (Cleveland Clinic 2020).

One type of dysautonomia that is frequently seen in Long COVID patients is POTS, a form of cardiac dysautonomia in which patients experience tachycardia (heart palpitations) and a rapid drop in blood pressure after moving into a standing position. POTS and dysautonomia can be extremely disruptive to an individual's ability to work and complete daily activities, with 60% of Long COVID patients with dysautonomia in one study being unable to return to work after eight months (Blitshteyn and Whitelaw 2021). Screening tools and tests for dysautonomia do exist, and many people with the condition improve with appropriate treatment (Dani et al. 2021). However, Long COVID patients may face barriers to receiving a correct diagnosis if their dysautonomia symptoms, such as tachycardia, are misdiagnosed as anxiety or a psychosomatic disorder.

2.3.3   Mast Cell Activation Syndrome (MCAS)

Mast Cell Activation Syndrome (MCAS) is a condition in which patients experience repeated anaphylactic episodes—including inflammation, itching, hives, and cardiac, respiratory, and gastrointestinal symptoms—with an unknown or seemingly nonexistent trigger (AAAAI 2022). These symptoms are caused by the activation of mast cells, which are typically responsible for the body's allergic response. MCAS and inflammation caused by persistent mast cell activation are believed to play a role in multiple autoimmune diseases, including rheumatoid arthritis and multiple sclerosis, due to the body's overly sensitive immune system attacking its own cells (Xu and Chen 2015).

Like ME/CFS, repeated instances of MCAS can permanently worsen the condition and result in higher baseline levels of inflammation and cytokine activity. Newly developed MCAS symptoms have been observed in a significant number of previously healthy Long COVID patients, with the symptoms experienced by these patients post-infection being nearly identical to those of MCAS patients with no history of COVID infection (Weinstock et al. 2021). Persistent immune activation and cytokine activity is a core component of the viral reservoir theory of Long COVID. This theory posits that the SARS-COV-2 virus infects and continues to replicate in some parts of the body such as nerve cells, the gastrointestinal tract, and adipose tissue after the acute illness has passed, leading to the over-active immune response seen in Long COVID patients (Buonsenso et al. 2022).

2.3.4   Small Fiber Neuropathy (SFN)

Small Fiber Neuropathy (SFN) is a condition caused by damage to peripheral nerves, causing symptoms such as numbness, pain, or burning sensations in the hands and feet. SFN is also associated with forms of autonomic dysfunction such as excessive sweating, dysfunctional temperature regulation, and cardiac dysregulation (Cleveland Clinic 2022). The nerve damage that occurs in SFN is believed to be autoimmune in nature. SFN is frequently comorbid with POTS, dysautonomia, and ME/CFS, and may contribute to their symptoms since damage to the connection between the Central Nervous System (CNS) and organ systems may reduce the CNS's ability to regulate the body's autonomic functions.

SFN is a common comorbidity in Long COVID and other IACIs (Abrams et al. 2022). One small study of Long COVID patients found that 60% of patients exhibited neuropathy based on three common diagnostic tests (Oaklander et al. 2022). SFN can be diagnosed through a skin biopsy, with the damage to peripheral nerves being visible on imaging studies (Fernandez et al. 2020). Other diagnostic tools include skin conductivity tests and autonomic function testing. These studies, combined with preexisting knowledge of the link between peripheral neuropathy and dysautonomia, have led some researchers to speculate that SFN contributes to disparate symptoms across organ systems experienced by some Long COVID patients.

2.3.5 Ehlers-Danlos Syndrome (EDS) and Hereditary Connective Tissue Disorders

Ehlers-Danlos Syndrome (EDS) is a family of hereditary connective tissue disorders involving mutations to the genes for collagen, a type of connective tissue found throughout the body. EDS commonly manifests as joint hypermobility, instability, or pain, but it is also noted for its extremely high rate of comorbidity with numerous systemic illnesses including chronic migraines, autonomic dysfunction, POTS, MCAS, ME/CFS, gastrointestinal symptoms, and neuropsychiatric conditions. One study of EDS patients with an average age of 36.7 years found that patients reported an average of 2.8 comorbid conditions (Song et al. 2020). Another study, which explored the relationship between hypermobility and ME/CFS, found that 41% of ME/CFS patients in the study met or exceeded the Beighton scale cutoff for joint hypermobility—compared to 3% of the general population (Bragee et al. 2020).

EDS is, perhaps mistakenly, considered a rare genetic disorder by many clinicians. Multiple facets of the disorder demonstrate that it is much more common than what diagnostic numbers indicate, and that it is a highly underdiagnosed condition rather than being a rare disorder. In children and teenagers, EDS tends to present as high joint flexibility—a trait that is often seen as benign and may even be advantageous for youth engaged in sports, dance, gymnastics, or other athletic activities. The numerous medical comorbidities associated with EDS only tend to manifest later in life, or after exposure to a trigger such as a viral infection (e.g., EBV/mononucleosis). As a result, patients with EDS are rarely screened for the disorder as children, and adults experiencing complex symptoms from the disorder are likely to have their symptoms attributed to other causes. A study of medical records in the United Kingdom (UK) found an average delay of 14 years between the first manifestation of EDS and its diagnosis, with 25% of patients waiting over 28 years for a diagnosis (Demmler et al. 2019). Over half of the patients surveyed in the study reported at least one misdiagnosis, and 86% of patients reported the diagnostic delay as being deleterious to their health.

The collagen mutations associated with EDS are perhaps the best-known example of a genetic risk factor for IACIs such as ME/CFS, dysautonomia, and Long COVID. Case studies of patients, often women in their 20–40 s, with joint hypermobility and experiencing extremely severe post-COVID symptoms after a mild acute infection have led some researchers to label the phenomenon as a sub-phenotype of post-COVID illness (Gavrilova et al. 2022). Other case studies, as well as anecdotal evidence from Long COVID patient groups, report the sudden manifestation of severe musculoskeletal disorders such as craniocervical instability (Barker et al. 2022), Chiari malformation (Espinoza et al. 2021), and Tethered Cord Syndrome (Mondal et al. 2021) after COVID-19 infection—indicating potentially severe interactions between COVID-19 infection and connective tissue within certain patients. EDS and other underdiagnosed connective tissue disorders represent a subset of people who are at extremely high risk for Long COVID—and who may be completely unaware of the risk that a COVID-19 infection poses to them.

2.3.6 IACIs Within Western Medicine

Infection-Associated Chronic Illnesses and related conditions are notorious for being among the most neglected and underfunded health conditions within Western medicine and science. Analysis of historical NIH funding of IACIs has found that ME/CFS research receives one of the lowest levels of funding from the NIH, relative to its prevalence, economic impact, and patients' quality of life. Prior to 2015, ME/CFS research received an average of $5 million in annual funding from the NIH. This number increased to $15 million per year after 2015, thanks to the National Academies' Institute of Medicine's ME/CFS report (IOM 2015). Even with this funding increase, it is estimated that ME/CFS research only receives about 7% of the funding of better-known illnesses with a similar level of disease burden (Miran et al. 2020). NIH funding of research on other IACIs and related conditions lags even behind ME/CFS—conditions such as MCAS and EDS have no record of NIH funding, and the first NIH funding for dysautonomia was for $2 million in 2020 (NIH RePORT 2023). This research gap for ME/CFS and related conditions exists similarly in clinical practice, with few dedicated specialists and FDA-approved treatments for these conditions.

The lack of basic research and clinical knowledge on IACIs is a major impediment to current action on Long COVID, but why does this extreme knowledge gap exist in the first place? IACIs' marginalization within Western science and medicine occurs primarily due to these illnesses not conforming to the standard practices and structures of these institutions. This mismatch manifests in multiple ways: two prominent ones being (1) the lack of a known biomarker for ME/CFS, Long COVID, and related conditions, and (2) the complex and multisystemic nature of IACIs placing them outside the scope of any one medical specialty.

Western medicine is structured around evidence-based practice, which uses objective measures and markers of disease to assign a diagnosis and guide treatment. Clinical approval for treatments requires multiple stages of clinical trials to demonstrate the safety and efficacy of new therapeutics. For the majority of illnesses and health conditions, evidence-based practice exists for a good reason—it ensures that diagnosis and treatment is backed up by scientific evidence, and that therapeutics have a measurable effect on a known disease process. However, many IACIs do not have a known biomarker, which severely hinders the ability of an evidence-based medical system to address these conditions.

The lack of biomarkers and definitive diagnostic tests for IACIs such as ME/CFS, fibromyalgia, and Long COVID means that from the perspective of Western medical practice, these illnesses are, at best, diagnoses of exclusion requiring extensive testing to rule out other potential causes of illness. However, many practitioners interpret IACIs' lack of known biomarkers to mean that there is no physiological basis for these illnesses, and that they are instead psychiatric or psychosomatic in nature. The complex and multi-systemic nature of IACIs can cause patients to experience a variety of seemingly-unrelated symptoms in different parts of the body, and there is little incentive on the part of any individual practitioner to spend time connecting the dots. The dynamics of the current medical system, in fact, encourage the exact opposite. Doctors are incentivized—if not required by their employer—to see as many patients as possible by spending a small amount of time with each individual patient, during which only their most pressing health issues are addressed. This makes it difficult for the underlying causes of complex illness to be correctly identified. This problem that is only made worse by a pre-existing lack of medical education on IACIs—only one-third of US medical schools in a 2013 survey covered ME/CFS in their curriculum (Peterson et al. 2013)—and the underfunding and short-staffing issues that are currently squeezing the healthcare system from all angles.

However, even patients who are able to obtain a proper diagnosis from their practitioner face significant hurdles to treatment from other parts of the healthcare system. With the lack of biomarkers comes a lack of clinically-approved treatments, meaning that therapeutics that may help alleviate symptoms must be prescribed off-label—a practice that is allowed, but disincentivized by standard medical practice. Insurance does not cover the cost of off-label prescriptions and treatments, so the expense of these treatments must be paid out-of-pocket. Few legal protections exist for practitioners who operate outside of an evidence base, so prescribing off-label treatments poses financial, legal, and professional risks for medical professionals. Unsurprisingly, many practitioners are unwilling to risk their license and professional reputation by prescribing experimental treatments for post-infectious and other complex chronic illnesses. The ones who do are often motivated by personal experience with this type of illness; such as being a caretaker for a family member or other loved one who is severely ill from a post-infectious condition, and having to navigate this bleak medical landscape on their behalf (Bateman 2023).

The lack of biomarkers for many types of multisystemic complex illness is ultimately a symptom of a much larger issue: these conditions have been deprioritized by Western medicine because they incompatible with how the medical system is structured. Medical care for serious forms of illness is handled by specialist practitioners. These providers operate within narrow domains of medicine that are delineated by organ systems—think of specialties and sub-specialties within fields such as cardiology, neurology, pulmonology, immunology, and so on. Specialists are experts at treating illnesses that lie within their domain, but have less expertise for medical issues that lie outside of their training. It is standard for specialists to refer patients out to other specialists for issues that they do not have the training to address on their own, or to work on a team with other specialists for complex illnesses with established treatment protocols, such as cancer.

However, complex multi-systemic illnesses such as IACIs are essentially homeless within this system: they exist at the margins of multiple medical specialties without being 'adopted' by any of them; have only a handful of dedicated experts that other practitioners can refer out to; and lack the research base and clinically-approved treatment protocols to allow for the development of interdisciplinary care teams (Bateman 2023). Complex illness patients seeking treatment often seek the care of multiple specialists—at no small cost—who address the symptoms that lie within their domain of expertise. There are few resources available to test for whether disparate illness symptoms being treated separately by different specialists may be linked to a single, non-obvious underlying cause.

The marginalization of IACIs and multi-systemic illnesses within science reflects the situation of these illnesses within medicine. Similar to how no medical specialty has adopted IACIs, these illnesses also have no obvious home within the NIH's research and funding structure. NIH funding that does exist for these illnesses is split primarily between the National Institutes for Allergy and Infectious Disease (NIAID) and National Institutes for Neurological Disorders and Stroke (NINDS), with studies occasionally being funded by a variety of smaller NIH bodies (NIH RePORT 2023). Although the bulk of the federal funding for IACI research comes from NIAID and NINDS, this money represents a very small fraction of the total budget for these large institutes. The bulk of the funding from these institutes goes towards well-known, high-priority diseases that lie clearly within their research domains, such as Alzheimer's Disease and stroke for NINDS, and HIV/AIDS, influenza, and emerging infectious diseases for NIAID. In order to receive funding from these large NIH institutes, IACI proposals must compete for attention against projects that are working off of a more substantial research base and are much closer to the institutes' core agenda (Spotila 2019). In this environment, only a handful of IACI funding requests make it through every year. As a result of this federal funding shortage, much of the IACI research base informing Long COVID research is funded through philanthropy and private sources.

The marginalization of IACIs and complex chronic illnesses within Western science and medicine is a vicious cycle. Decades of research under-investment has created significant gaps in medical field's understanding of these diseases, and perhaps most crucially, has left practitioners without objective biomarkers on which to base diagnosis and treatment. These research gaps have caused IACIs to be given minimal attention in medical education curricula, resulting in many practitioners not being trained to handle this type of complex illness. Doctors are further disincentivized from devoting large amounts of time to any one patient's case, and may be seriously penalized for working outside of standard protocols, such as prescribing off-label medications or experimental therapies for illnesses that have few-to-no clinically-approved treatments. The larger healthcare and research systems are not well set up to accommodate IACIs en masse, due to these illnesses exhibiting fundamental conflicts with the existing structure of these systems. Future progress on IACIs will likely require new, interdisciplinary approaches to research and treatment—which the scale of complex disability caused by COVID may be significant enough to catalyze.

2.3.7   Discussion

The challenges faced by people with ME/CFS and other complex chronic conditions—in terms of physiological symptoms, interactions with medical providers and insurers, and broader social impacts—are a preview of the risks being faced by people with Long COVID. More specifically, they are a preview of the risks people with Long COVID will face if the current status quo is maintained. In terms of physiological symptoms, Long COVID is not a new or unique condition. It has considerable overlap with other post-infectious syndromes and may ultimately represent an expansion of this type of disease burden.

However, Long COVID differs from other IACIs in one crucial way: the illness is definitively linked to the COVID-19 pandemic, a specific and highly publicized event that has disrupted nearly all aspects of daily life around the world. This distinction is important for recognizing Long COVID as a medical condition as proving causality between a previous viral infection and lingering ill-health is a major barrier to diagnosing post-infectious illness.

People with ME/CFS and other IACIs have long struggled to have their illnesses recognized—both by their medical providers and by the communities and systems that they rely on for support and survival, in part because their symptoms are difficult to attribute to any one cause or event. With the emergence of Long COVID, this conversation is starting to change—partly because the COVID-19 pandemic has become a focusing event for millions of people newly disabled by Long COVID, and millions more who have been living with neglected complex chronic illness for years.

2.4   The Long-Hauler Movement

During the chaos of the early years of the COVID-19 pandemic, healthcare systems and governments around the world struggled to manage the exponential spread of the virus and its overwhelming of emergency rooms and ICUs. Although only a fraction of people infected with the virus developed symptoms severe enough to warrant hospitalization, the volume of people infected combined with the complex care and slow recovery of hospitalized COVID patients was enough to focus nearly all medical, political, and media attention on the acute crisis.

COVID-19 was portrayed as a disease with a dichotomous outcome—people either experienced a flu-like illness and eventually recovered or became severely ill and were at risk for a slow, suffocating, isolated death. Severe illness was most commonly associated with age or the presence of underlying health conditions. The characteristics of acute COVID-19 observed during the early pandemic set the stage for the dominant narrative around the virus's risk profile—elderly and disabled people were at the highest risk for severe disease and death, and while the rest of the population should act to avoid infecting the medically vulnerable, they were not personally at great risk from the virus.

However, this dominant narrative did not reflect the reality that many people who had been infected in the early months of the pandemic were experiencing. Instead of recovering to a state of normal health after their initial infection, these patients experienced months of debilitating symptoms such as difficulty breathing, fatigue, and neurological problems. With no acknowledgment of these symptoms coming from the medical community, advisory agencies such as the CDC, or the media, COVID survivors turned to the Internet for answers and found out they were far from alone. The phenomenon of Long COVID was identified and self-named by "Long-Haulers" connecting with each other over social media platforms such as Facebook. The widespread shift to online forms of communication during the early pandemic lockdowns not only enabled long-haulers to corroborate their experiences with each other, but also to connect with COVID survivors from European countries that had experienced early COVID waves and members of other chronic illness communities (Callard and Perego 2021). The name "Long COVID" was first used in May 2020, and by July and August 2020, the medical community and some members of the press began to investigate this new condition that defied common media portrayals of COVID-19.

The long-hauler community's pressure on official information channels to acknowledge their condition, as well as their patient-directed research to document the illness profile and trajectory of Long COVID, has played a crucial role in this new illness being legitimized by medical authorities. As the pandemic has progressed and the picture and scale of Long COVID become clearer, more research on the illness is being conducted, often in collaboration with long-hauler groups. However, as a 2021 expose by science writer Ed Yong explores, uncertainty remains about the future of Long COVID and whether long-haulers will be able to maintain their initial position of expertise over their illness (Yong 2021).

The question of who holds the expertise—between patients with lived experience and doctors with medical training and authority—is a source of tension in many areas of medical research. Additional concerns have been raised about how the experiences and needs of long-haulers come into conflict with dominant political and economic narratives surrounding COVID that present the pandemic as a temporary problem and encourage a rapid return to the pre-pandemic status quo. As the rest of society catches up to the reality of Long COVID, many questions remain about what the future holds for people who caught COVID-19 and never fully recovered.

2.5   Current Policy Approaches

The grassroots Long COVID advocacy movement has been remarkably successful in drawing the attention of the medical, research, and policy communities, with Long COVID being recognized as a serious medical condition as early as 2020. However, significant challenges remain in translating awareness of Long COVID into concrete policy action—particularly when it comes to changes that meaningfully address the lives of long haulers. Current policy approaches to this issue in the United States include the NIH's RECOVER initiative, the introduction of several Congressional bills to increase Long COVID education and awareness, and the establishment of Long COVID clinics by hospital systems across the country.

2.5.1   NIH and the RECOVER Initiative

The primary policy action that the US federal government has taken to address Long COVID is the allocation of research money to the National Institutes of Health (NIH) to study the condition. Nearly all of the NIH's Long COVID funding is allocated to the RECOVER Initiative—a multidisciplinary Long COVID research program that was established in September 2020, and later expanded with $1.15 billion from Congress in February 2021 (Subbaraman 2021). The RECOVER Initiative has been described as a "slow-moving glacier"—an ambitious project with a goal of recruiting 40,000 participants at over 30 institutions across the US (Cohrs 2022). However, progress on achieving the study's recruitment goals has been slow, and a perceived lack of urgency and progress has drawn the ire of some Long COVID patient groups.

The goal of the RECOVER Initiative is to fund studies that investigate the following questions:

1. What is the clinical spectrum of, and the biology underlying recovery from, acute SARS-CoV-2 infection over time?
2. For those patients who do not fully recover, what is the incidence/prevalence, natural history, clinical spectrum, and underlying biology of this condition? Are there distinct phenotypes of patients who have prolonged symptoms or other sequelae?
3. Does SARS-CoV-2 infection initiate or promote the pathogenesis of conditions or findings that evolve to cause organ dysfunction or increase the risk of developing other disorders?

The task of building a robust network of Long COVID researchers is complicated—due in part to the complex nature of the disease itself and medicine's past failures to adequately address multi-systemic illness. Because Long COVID can impact numerous bodily systems, RECOVER has recruited experts from many different medical specialties, who often require supplemental education on aspects of Long COVID that lie outside of their area of expertise. This learning curve is made more difficult by a dearth of multidisciplinary medical expertise and specialists who focus on complex multisystem illnesses such as ME/CFS, dysautonomia, MCAS, and other post-infectious illnesses that overlap with Long COVID and have historically received little research funding. In many cases, experts involved with RECOVER have had little prior exposure to post-infectious illnesses, and must be brought up to speed on the existing body of knowledge on these conditions (Bateman 2023). Having to lay the groundwork to conduct large-scale studies on a complex illness requiring interdisciplinary knowledge and cooperation has hindered RECOVER's ability to launch quickly.

RECOVER's progress has also been slowed by much lower patient recruitment numbers than originally inticipated. As of 2022, NIH reported that only 3% of the intended 40,000 study participants had been recruited—baffling observers both within and outside of NIH (Cohrs 2022). Numerous explanations for the recruitment shortage have been put forth: including unclear instructions on how patients can find a study site and register for the program, a lack of communication with interested participants who have registered, and exclusion criteria that deem some Long COVID patients—such as people who were infected over a year ago—ineligible for certain studies.

However, perhaps the most important explanation for RECOVER's recruitment problems—and a major criticism of the program from patient advocates—is that many Long COVID patients have little extra time and energy to devote to observational studies that do not offer anything in the way of potential treatments. This split between the priorities of the scientific and patient communities illustrates one of the main conflicts at the heart of Long COVID research. From a scientific perspective, collecting robust observational data from a large cohort of patients experiencing a novel illness is an extremely valuable source of knowledge, with long-term potential to inform future studies and treatments for post-infectious illnesses. However, what this framework fails to take into consideration is that many Long COVID patients are struggling to merely survive with debilitating symptoms, limited energy, and increasingly dire economic hardships.

The COVID-19 Long-Hauler Advocacy Project (C-19 LAP), a patient-led research group, conducted a survey of the economic burden of Long COVID in 2021. Their survey found that in addition to high medical bills (an average of over $17,000 per person in the sample), nearly half of the long-haulers surveyed were completely unable to work, and the other half were working at partial capacity. Only 5% of the sample reported being able to work at full capacity (C-19 LAP 2021). Some people experiencing Long COVID are able to access short-term forms of financial support, such as relying on family or applying for short-term disability programs, but significantly fewer economic support options are available for medium-to-long-term disability. Long-haulers also face significant restrictions on their available time and energy due to their newfound health problems, with those experiencing ME/CFS symptoms such as fatigue and post-exertional malaise being unable to take on additional activity without risking a worsening of their condition.

Observational research studies, such as the large one being put together by RECOVER, typically do not confer any personal benefit to participants. This is in contrast to clinical trial studies, which offer the possibility of symptom alleviation through experimental treatment. For a typical study population, the lack of personal benefit is not an issue, since the risk undertaken by participants is generally also small-to-nonexistent. This is a key way in which Long COVID patients differ from typical patient populations. Because of the severe health challenges and dire economic straits that many Long Haulers experience, participation in a research study may result in harmful externalities that a typical patient population would not experience. Critics of the RECOVER Initiative's approach argue that the study's slow, "business-as-usual" pace fails to realize the urgency of Long COVID—especially when the rapid response to the acute COVID crisis and the swift development of the COVID vaccine in the earlier stages of the pandemic demonstrate what sort of innovation is possible when given sufficient funding and willpower (Ladyzhets 2022).

The RECOVER Initiative's slow progress has drawn criticism from patient advocate groups, and the NIH's lack of transparency surrounding the project has not helped the situation. Although nearly all of RECOVER's funding is allocated internally, the NIH has been slow to release details on what specific projects the initiative will fund. Given that practically all of the federal research money for Long COVID is allocated to RECOVER, this has raised fears among patient advocates already critical of the program that this once-in-a-lifetime opportunity to crack the mysteries of long-neglected complex illnesses could be squandered by a bureaucratic system that fails to realize the urgency of the problem that it is being tasked with solving. Other concerns raised by RECOVER's slow progress are the possibility that no additional funding will be provided for the initiative if COVID falls from the political agenda; and the fact that as the virus continues to spread, it will become difficult to design studies examining the long-term impacts of infection as the number of people who have never been infected dwindles. This could make it challenging to establish a true control group to compare the increasingly common outcomes of infection to.

2.5.2 Congressional Action

In addition to the research funding allocated by Congress to the NIH to study Long COVID, the conversations about long-term disability stirred up by the pandemic have led to several bills that would address the needs of long-haulers and others living with disabilities. Patient advocates helped craft and advocate for the COVID-19 Long Haulers Act, which would authorize $63 million in Long COVID research for the Patient-Centered Outcomes Research Institute (PCORI), Agency of Healthcare Quality and Research (AHRQ), and Centers for Medicare and Medicaid Services (CMS), as well as $30 million to the CDC for outreach and education about Long COVID to medical providers and the general public (Solve 2021).

The pandemic has also renewed advocacy to increase funding for Home and Community-Based Services (HBCS). The COVID HCBS Relief Act of 2021 was introduced to temporarily increase Medicaid funding for home-based care, and a $150 billion expansion and strengthening of Medicaid HBCS was included in the November 2021 Build Back Better bill (Aguilar 2021)—but significantly scaled back in the final legislation. A broader bill that has been introduced in Congress to address the needs of people with disabilities is the Supplemental Security Income (SSI) Restoration Act of 2021. This bill would fix many problems with SSI that disability rights advocates have long sought to fix—including the failure to adjust payments for inflation and cost-of-living increases, a $2,000 asset limit, and the termination of disability benefits for married individuals (US Congress 2021; Buffie 2021).

In March of 2022, the Government Accountability Office (GAO) released a report estimating that between 7 and 23 million Americans could be living with Long COVID—based on the number of reported COVID cases and a Long COVID prevalence range of 10–30% of survivors (GAO 2022). This report led multiple members of Congress to release statements calling for more action on Long COVID—including Senator Tim Kaine of Virginia, who was the first member of Congress to publicly admit having Long COVID symptoms (Ollstein 2022). Other members of Congress, such as Senator Sheldon Whitehouse, have released inquiries into the federal government's Long COVID response to agencies such as the NIH and SSA office (Whitehouse and Markey 2022; Whitehouse 2022). However, nearly all congressional advocacy on Long COVID has come from Democratic members of Congress—in the climate of this government body being highly polarized and evenly split between Democrats and Republicans. In the absence of GOP support or acknowledgment, all existing pieces of Long COVID legislation remain stalled in Congress.

2.5.3   Post-COVID Clinics

Some hospitals, healthcare systems, and universities have worked to address the needs of long-haulers through the establishment of post-COVID clinics. Post-COVID clinics leverage existing healthcare networks to evaluate the individual needs of long-haulers, who can present with a range of symptoms and symptom clusters, and refer them to specialists associated with the network (Walter 2021). This system can make the process of addressing the medical needs of long-haulers more efficient and can save them the stress of having to find specialists who are knowledgeable about Long COVID on their own.

However, the demand for post-COVID clinics far exceeds the supply—many of these clinics have months-long waiting lists for an initial evaluation, and even after this initial evaluation, patients may continue to experience delayed treatment due to specialist waiting lists. Additionally, most existing post-COVID clinics are run by large hospital systems and universities and rely on healthcare networks in urban areas—a barrier to care for rural post-COVID patients. The lack of centralization and standardization for post-COVID clinics causes the level of care and available programs offered at each site to vary—with Long COVID patients reporting relatively little substantial help being offered by some clinics.

When the Threatcasting workshop was run in August 2021, concrete policy action on Long COVID was stalled by a lack of official diagnostic criteria for Long COVID and a lack of research into the underlying causes of the disease. In the year since, progress has been made in many of these areas—diagnostic criteria have been clarified, and research on multiple potential biomarkers and disease processes for Long COVID has been published. However, uptake of these advances remains imperfect, since many medical practitioners remain undereducated about Long COVID, clinical trials are progressing slowly, and biomarker research has yet to translate into clinically-applicable treatments. One shortcoming of focusing on Long COVID policy through a medicalized lens is that it risks reducing Long COVID to a medical problem whose solutions lie at the level of the individual. As data on the individual and societal economic impacts of Long COVID exemplify, the macro-level impacts of COVID-19 as a mass-disabling event go far beyond any one individual or field of study. To truly conceptualize and address the full impact of Long COVID, a stronger interdisciplinary and systems-level approach is needed.

References

AAAAI (2022) Mast Cell Activation Syndrome (MCAS). American Academy of Allergy, Asthma & Immunology. https://www.aaaai.org/conditions-treatments/related-conditions/mcas. Accessed 20 Sept 2022

Abrams R, Simpson D, Navis A et al (2022) Small fiber neuropathy associated with SARS-CoV-2 infection. Mus Ner. 65:440–443. https://doi.org/10.1002/mus.27458

Aguilar E (2021) The build back better act: $150 billion for medicaid HCBS funding and other important programs. American Network of Community Options and Resources. https://www.ancor.org/newsroom/news/build-back-better-act-150-billion-medicaid-hcbs-funding-and-other-important-programs. Accessed 20 Jan 2022

Al-Aly Z, Xie Y, Bowe B (2021) High-dimensional characterization of post-acute sequelae of COVID-19. Nature 594:259–264. https://doi.org/10.1038/s41586-021-03553-9

Allen J, Almukhtar S, Aufrichtig A et al. (2021). Coronavirus in the U.S.: Latest Map and Case Count. New York Times. https://www.nytimes.com/interactive/2021/us/covid-cases.html. Accessed 20 Jan 2022

Araja D, Berkis U, Lunga A, Murovska M (2021) Shadow Burden of Undiagnosed Myalgic Encephalomyelitis/Chronic Fatigue Syndrome (ME/CFS) on Society: Retrospective and Prospective—In Light of COVID-19. J. Clin. Med. https://doi.org/10.3390/jcm10143017

Asbring P, Narvanen AL (2003) Ideal versus reality: Physicians perspectives on patients with chronic fatigue syndrome (CFS) and fibromyalgia. Social Science & Medicine 57:711–720

Asbring P (2001) Chronic illness—a disruption in life: identity-transformation among women with chronic fatigue syndrome and fibromyalgia. J Adv Nurs. 34:312–9. https://doi.org/10.1046/j.1365-2648.2001.01767.x

Ayoubkhani D, Nafilyan V, Humberstone B, Banerjee A (2021) Post-COVID syndrome in individuals admitted to hospital with COVID-19: Retrospective cohort study. BMJ. https://doi.org/10.1136/bmj.n693

Baig A, Khaleeq A, Syeda H (2020) Elucidation of cellular targets and exploitation of the receptor-binding domain of SARS-CoV-2 for vaccine and monoclonal antibody synthesis. J Med Vir 92:2792–2803. https://doi.org/10.1002/jmv.26212

Barker S, Mujallid R, Bayanzay K (2022) Atlantoaxial subluxation secondary to SARS-COV-2 infection: A rare orthopedic complication from COVID-19. Am J Case Rep. https://doi.org/10.12659/ajcr.936128

Bateman L (2023) Personal Communication. May 19, 2023.

Bayliss K, Riste L, Fisher L et al (2014) Diagnosis and management of chronic fatigue syndrome/myalgic encephalitis in black and minority ethnic people: a qualitative study. Prim Health Care Res Dev. 15:143–55. https://doi.org/10.1017/S1463423613000145

Blease C, Geraghty K (2018) Are ME/CFS patient organizations militant? J Bio Inq 15:396–40. https://doi.org/10.1007/s11673-018-9866-5

Blitshteyn S, Whitelaw S (2021) Postural orthostatic tachycardia syndrome (POTS) and other autonomic disorders after COVID-19 infection: A case series of 20 patients. Immunol Res. 69:205–211. https://doi.org/10.1007/s12026-021-09185-5

Bonilla H, Quach TC, Tiwari A et al (2022) Myalgic encephalomyelitis/chronic fatigue syndrome (ME/CFS) is common in post-acute sequelae of SARS-CoV-2 infection (PASC): Results from a post-COVID-19 multidisciplinary clinic. MedRxiv. https://doi.org/10.1101/2022.08.03.22278363

Bougakov D, Podell K, Goldberg E (2021) Multiple neuroinvasive pathways in COVID-19. Mol Neu 58:564–575. https://doi.org/10.1007/s12035-020-02152-5

Bragee B, Michos A, Drum B et al (2020) Signs of intracranial hypertension, hypermobility, and craniocervical obstructions in patients with myalgic encephalomyelitis/chronic fatigue syndrome. Front. Neurol. https://doi.org/10.3389/fneur.2020.00828

Buffie N (2021) SSI reform would boost incomes for seniors and disabled people. Center for American Progress. https://www.americanprogress.org/article/ssi-reform-boost-incomes-seniors-disabled-people/. Accessed 20 Jan 2022

Buonsenso D, Piazza M, Boner A et al (2022) Long COVID: A proposed hypothesis-driven model of viral persistence for the pathophysiology of the syndrome. Allergy Asthma Proc. 43:187–193. https://doi.org/10.2500/aap.2022.43.220018

Burrell C, Howard C, Murphy F (2017) Viral syndromes. Fenner and White's Medical Virology. 2017:537–556. https://doi.org/10.1016/b978-0-12-375156-0.00039-4

C-19 LAP (2021) Mathematical breakdown and formulas for long COVID calculations. COVID-19 Longhauler Advocacy Project. https://www.longhauler-advocacy.org/calculations-formulas

Callard F, Perego E (2021) How and why patients made long COVID. Soc Sci Med. https://doi.org/10.1016/j.socscimed.2020.113426

CDC (2021) Interim clinical guidance for management of patients with confirmed coronavirus disease (COVID-19) Centers for Disease Control and Prevention. https://www.cdc.gov/coronavirus/2019-ncov/hcp/clinical-guidance-management-patients.html. Accessed 20 Jan 2022

CDC (2022) Nearly one in five American adults who have had COVID-19 still have long COVID. Centers for Disease Control and Prevention. https://www.cdc.gov/nchs/pressroom/nchs_press_r eleases/2022/20220622.htm. Accessed 20 Sept 2022

Chung T, Mastalerz MH, Morrow AK et al (2021) COVID long haulers: Long-term effects of COVID-19. https://www.hopkinsmedicine.org/health/conditions-and-diseases/coronavirus/ covid-long-haulers-long-term-effects-of-covid19. Accessed 20 Jan 2022

Cleveland Clinic (2020) Dysautonomia. Cleveland Clinic. https://my.clevelandclinic.org/health/dis eases/6004-dysautonomia. Accessed 20 Jan 2022

Cleveland Clinic (2022) Cutaneous Nerve Laboratory. Cleveland Clinic. https://my.clevelandclinic. org/health/diagnostics/16905-cutaneous-nerve-laboratory. Accessed 20 Sept 2022

Cohrs R (2022) 'A slow-moving glacier': NIH's sluggish and often opaque efforts to study long Covid draw patient, expert ire. STAT News. https://www.statnews.com/2022/03/29/nih-long-covid-sluggish-study/

Dani M, Dirksen A, Taraborrelli P (2021) Autonomic dysfunction in 'long COVID': rationale, physiology and management strategies. Clin Med (Lond). 2:63–67. https://doi.org/10.7861/clinmed.2020-0896

Davis H, Assaf G, McCorkill L et al (2021) Characterizing long COVID in an international cohort: 7 months of symptoms and their impact. eClin Med 38:1–19. https://doi.org/10.1016/j.eclinm.2021.101019

Demmler J, Atkinson M, Reinhold E (2019) Diagnosed prevalence of ehlers-danlos syndrome and hypermobility spectrum disorder in Wales, UK: A national electronic cohort study and case–control comparison. BMJ Open. https://doi.org/10.1136/bmjopen-2019-031365

Dowdy D, D'Souza G (2020) COVID-19 testing: Understanding the percent positive. Johns Hopkins Bloomberg School of Public Health. https://publichealth.jhu.edu/2020/covid-19-testing-und erstanding-the-percent-positive

Dunne P, Smallwood M, Taylor E (2022) Long COVID impact on adult Americans: early indicators estimating prevalence and cost. Solve long COVID Initiative. https://solvecfs.org/wp-content/upl oads/2022/04/long_covid_impact_paper.pdf. Accessed 20 Sept 2022

Eaton-Fitch N, Johnston SC, Zalewski P et al (2020) Health-related quality of life in patients with myalgic encephalomyelitis/chronic fatigue syndrome: an Australian cross-sectional study. Qual Life Res. 2020; 29:1521–1531. https://doi.org/10.1007/s11136-019-02411-6

Espinoza J, Junior J, Miranda C (2021) Atypical COVID–19 presentation with budd-chiari syndrome leading to an outbreak in the emergency department. Am J Emerg Med 46:800.e5–800.e7. https://doi.org/10.1016/j.ajem.2021.01.090

Fernandez C, Franz C, Ko J et al (2020) Imaging review of peripheral nerve injuries in patients with COVID-19. Radiology. https://doi.org/10.1148/radiol.2020203116

GAO (2022) Science & tech spotlight: Long COVID. U.S. Government Accountability Office. https://www.gao.gov/products/gao-22-105666. Accessed 20 Sept 2022

Gavrilova N, Soprun L, Lukashenko M et al (2022) New clinical phenotype of the post-COVID syndrome: fibromyalgia and joint hypermobility condition. Pathophysiology 2022, 29:24–29. https://doi.org/10.3390/pathophysiology29010003

Gold J, Okyay R, Licht W et al (2021) Investigation of long COVID prevalence and its relationship to epstein-barr virus reactivation. Pathogens. https://doi.org/10.3390/pathogens10060763

Guise J, McVittie C, McKinlay A (2010) A discourse analytic study of ME/CFS (chronic fatigue syndrome) sufferers' experiences of interactions with doctors. J Hea Psy. https://doi.org/10.1177/1359105309350515

Huang Y, Pinto M, Borelli J et al (2022) COVID symptoms, symptom clusters, and predictors for becoming a long-hauler: Looking for clarity in the haze of the pandemic. Clin Nur Res. https://doi.org/10.1177/10547738221125632

Institute of Medicine (2015) Beyond myalgic encephalomyelitis/chronic fatigue syndrome: redefining an illness. Washington, DC: The National Academies Press. https://doi.org/10.17226/19012

Ladyzhets B (2022) The U.S. has had the most COVID cases in the world. Why isn't it doing more to study long COVID? Grid News. https://www.grid.news/story/science/2022/05/09/the-us-has-had-the-most-covid-cases-in-the-world-why-isnt-it-doing-more-to-study-long-covid/. Accessed 20 Sept 2022

Larsen N, Stiles L, Shaik R (2022) Characterization of autonomic symptom burden in long COVID: A global survey of 2,314 adults. MedRxiv. https://doi.org/10.1101/2022.04.25.22274300

Mancini D, Brunjes D, Lala A et al (2021) Use of Cardiopulmonary stress testing for patients with unexplained dyspnea post–coronavirus disease. J Am Coll Cardiol HF. 20219: 927–937. https://doi.org/10.1016/j.jchf.2021.10.002

Miran A, Dimmock M, Jason L (2020). Research update: The relation between ME/CFS disease burden and research funding in the USA. Work. https://content.iospress.com/articles/work/wor203173#ref001%20ref008%20ref009

Mondal R, Deb S, Shome G et al (2021) COVID-19 and emerging spinal cord complications: A systematic review. Mult Scler Relat Disord. https://doi.org/10.1016/j.msard.2021.102917

NASEM (2023) Toward a Common Research Agenda in Infection-Associated Chronic Illnesses: A Workshop to Examine Common, Overlapping Clinical and Biological Factors. National Academies of Science, Engineering, and Medicine. https://www.nationalacademies.org/our-work/toward-a-common-research-agenda-in-infection-associated-chronic-illnesses-a-workshop-to-examine-common-overlapping-clinical-and-biological-factors. Accessed 30 May 2023.

NIH (2011) Myalgic encephalomyelitis/chronic fatigue syndrome (me/cfs) research: Workshop Report. National Institutes of Health. https://meassociation.org.uk/wp-content/uploads/2011/08/sok-workshop-report-508-compliant-8-5-11.pdf

NIH RePORT (2023) Estimates of Funding for Various Research, Condition, and Disease Categories (RCDC). National Institutes of Health. https://report.nih.gov/funding/categorical-spending/

Oaklander AL, Mills A, Kelley M et al (2022) Peripheral neuropathy evaluations of patients with prolonged long COVID. Neurol Neuroimmunol Neuroinflamm. https://doi.org/10.1212/NXI.0000000000001146

Ollstein A (2022) Tim Kaine has long COVID. That's not moving congress to act. Politico. https://www.politico.com/news/2022/08/08/long-covid-congress-kaine-00049921. Accessed 20 Sept 2022

Patterson B, Guevara-Coto J, Yogendra R et al (2021) Immune-based prediction of COVID-19 severity and chronicity decoded using machine learning. Frontiers in Immunology. https://doi.org/10.3389/fimmu.2021.700782

Pendergrast T, Brown A, Sunnquist M et al (2016) Housebound versus nonhousebound patients with myalgic encephalomyelitis and chronic fatigue syndrome. Chr Illn 12:292–307. https://doi.org/10.1177/1742395316644770

Peterson, TM, Peterson TW, Emerson S, Regalbuto E, Evans MA, Jason LA (2013) Coverage of CFS within U.S. Medical Schools. Universal Journal of Public Health, 1(4), 177–179. https://doi.org/10.13189/ujph.2013.010404.

PHOSP-COVID Collaborative Group et al (2021) Physical, cognitive and mental health impacts of COVID-19 following hospitalization: A multi-centre prospective cohort study. MedRxiv. https://doi.org/10.1101/2021.03.22.21254057

Pretorius E, Vlok M, Bezuidenhout J et al (2021) Persistent clotting protein pathology in long COVID/post-acute sequelae of COVID-19 (pasc) is accompanied by increased levels of antiplasmin. Cardiovascular Diabetology. https://doi.org/10.1186/s12933-021-01359-7

Rahmandad H, Lim T, Sterman J (2021) Behavioral dynamics of COVID-19: estimating under-reporting, multiple waves, and adherence fatigue across 92 nations. System Dynamics Review (Forthcoming). https://doi.org/10.2139/ssrn.3635047

Sah P, Fitzpatrick M, Zimmer C et al (2021) Asymptomatic SARS-CoV-2 infection: A systematic review and meta-analysis. PNAS 118 (34). https://doi.org/10.1073/pnas.2109229118

Scialo F, Daniele A, Amato F et al (2020) ACE2: The major cell entry receptor for SARS-COV-2. Lung. 198:867–877. https://doi.org/10.1007/s00408-020-00408-4

Seeßle J, Waterboer T, Hippchen T et al (2021) Persistent symptoms in adult patients 1 year after coronavirus disease 2019 (COVID-19): A prospective cohort study. Clin Infect Dis. https://doi.org/10.1093/cid/ciab611

Shear M, Goodnough A, Kaplan S et al (2021) The lost month: how a failure to test blinded the U.S. to COVID-19. New York Times. https://www.nytimes.com/2020/03/28/us/testing-coronavirus-pandemic.html. Accessed 20 Sept 2022

SMA (2021) An Overview of Post-viral Syndrome. Southern Medical Association. https://sma.org/post-viral-syndrome/

Solve ME (2021) The COVID-19 longhaulers act. Solve ME/CFS Initiative. https://solvecfs.org/wp-content/uploads/2021/04/covid-19-longhaulers-act-1pg-final.pdf

Song B, Yeh P, Harrel J (2020) Systemic manifestations of ehlers-danlos syndrome. Proc (Bayl Univ Med Cent). 2021 Jan; 34:49–53. https://doi.org/10.1080/08998280.2020.1805714

Spotila J (2019) The NIH is thwarting research on a poorly understood yet serious condition. StatNews. https://www.statnews.com/2019/01/10/nih-obstacles-thwart-myalgic-encephalomyelitis-research/. Accessed 5 June 2023.

Subbaraman N (2021) US health agency will invest $1 billion to investigate 'long COVID'. Nature. https://www.nature.com/articles/d41586-021-00586-y. Accessed 20 Jan 2022

Taquet M, Dercon Q, Luciano S et al (2021) Incidence, co-occurrence, and evolution of long-COVID features: A 6-month retrospective cohort study of 273,618 survivors of COVID-19. PLOS Med. https://doi.org/10.1371/journal.pmed.1003773

Thaweethai T, Jolley S, Karlson E et al (2023) Development of a Definition of Postacute Sequelae of SARS-CoV-2 Infection. JAMA. https://doi.org/10.1001/jama.2023.8823

US Congress (2021) Text - S.2065 - 117th Congress (2021–2022): Supplemental security income restoration act of 2021. http://www.congress.gov/. Accessed 20 Dec 2021

Utah Long-Haulers Patient Group (2022) What cognitive dysfunction looks like for many COVID long-haulers. Private Communication, 2022, Sept 17

Walter K (2021) An inside look at a post–COVID-19 clinic. JAMA. https://jamanetwork.com/journals/jama/fullarticle/2779851. Accessed 20 Jan 2022

Wang X, Zhou Y, Jiang N et al (2020) Persistence of intestinal SARS-CoV-2 infection in patients with COVID-19 leads to re-admission after pneumonia resolved. Int J Infect Dis. 2020 Jun; 95: 433–435. doi: https://doi.org/10.1016/j.ijid.2020.04.063

Weinstock L, Brook J, Walters A (2021) Mast cell activation symptoms are prevalent in long-COVID. Int J Infect Dis. 112:217–226. https://doi.org/10.1016/j.ijid.2021.09.043

Whitehouse S (2022) SSA long COVID letter. Office of senator Sheldon Whitehouse. https://www.whitehouse.senate.gov/imo/media/doc/final%20ssa%20long%20covid%20letter.pdf. Accessed 20 Sept 2022

Wiech M, Chroscicki P, Swatler J et al (2022) Remodeling of T cell dynamics during long COVID is dependent on severity of SARS-CoV-2 infection. Frontiers in Immunology. https://doi.org/10.3389/fimmu.2022.886431

World Health Organization (WHO) (2021). WHO coronavirus (COVID-19) dashboard. https://covid19.who.int. Accessed 20 June 2022

Xu Y, Chen G (2015) Mast cell and autoimmune diseases. Mediators Inflamm. https://doi.org/10.1155/2015/246126

Yong E (2021) Long-haulers are fighting for their future. The Atlantic. https://www.theatlantic.com/science/archive/2021/09/covid-19-long-haulers-pandemic-future/619941/

International Perspectives on Long COVID

3

In October 2021, the World Health Organization (WHO) released its clinical definition of post COVID-19 condition—also known as Long COVID or Post-Acute Sequelae of COVID-19 (PASC). The WHO's guidance describes this condition as:

> Post COVID-19 condition occurs in individuals with a history of probable or confirmed SARS CoV-2 infection, usually 3 months from the onset of COVID-19 with symptoms and that last for at least 2 months and cannot be explained by an alternative diagnosis. Common symptoms include fatigue, shortness of breath, cognitive dysfunction but also others and generally have an impact on everyday functioning. Symptoms may be new onset following initial recovery from an acute COVID-19 episode or persist from the initial illness. Symptoms may also fluctuate or relapse over time. (WHO 2021)

The WHO's release of an official definition of Long COVID was a valuable and long-awaited step in the official acknowledgement of this illness. The WHO's announcement gave medical professionals and policymakers an official document from a trusted global health organization that they could point to regarding the reality of this problem. Other public health bodies, such as the US's CDC released their own interim guidance on Long COVID shortly after the release of the WHO's consensus definition. This increased awareness of the condition among medical practitioners, policymakers, and the general public, and opened the door to further discussion on how to address Long COVID globally. However, the question remained: How much would the WHO's guidance actually go on to influence policy action?

The global nature of the COVID-19 pandemic means that Long COVID and other forms of post-COVID disability will impact nearly every country in the world—regardless of the capacity of local health systems to handle this surge of new disability. From its inception, COVID research and the Long COVID patient movement have been international efforts facilitated by social media and other online platforms, enabling collaboration and information-sharing with little regard for physical distance or international borders. Global teams conducting COVID and Long COVID research on patient cohorts across the world have greatly accelerated knowledge collection about this new disease.

Population-level analysis of post-COVID conditions from countries with the healthcare infrastructure to collect this data has aided the characterization and prevalence estimates in countries that lack this infrastructure. However, despite the universality of COVID-19 and its sequelae, the reality of treatment and the intersection of post-COVID disability with other sociopolitical factors may differ widely in different regions of the world. When thinking about the long-term impact of COVID-19 and its intersections with complex sociopolitical systems, it is important to consider how post-COVID disability may present itself and affect communities outside of the US, and the outcomes that this may have in conjunction with other geopolitical factors.

This chapter offers an overview of Long COVID around the world, and how the pandemic response of countries outside of the US impacted the trajectories of people living with post-COVID medical complications. This perspective was missing from the Long COVID Threatcasting pilot project, which focused on the US, its institutions, and the aspects of American healthcare and social safety nets that set it apart from much of the rest of the world.

As of 2022, significant gaps remain in the ability of healthcare and economic support systems around the world to meet the needs of post-COVID patients due to a lack of approved treatments for complex and severe forms of the illness, as well as shortages of healthcare resources and workers. Most of the attention on Long COVID has come from wealthier Western countries such as the US, the UK, and continental Europe—which are simultaneously global scientific leaders, and which have had substantially higher numbers of COVID cases than most other regions of the world due to policies that failed to control the pandemic.

In Western countries with high case rates, Long COVID has entered the political conversation primarily due to its impact on the labor force and its role in causing ongoing high job vacancy levels. Government and media acknowledgment of Long COVID exists in competition with broader narratives on the pandemic that encourage the lifting of COVID mitigations and a "return to normalcy"—regardless of the contradictions between these two adjacent narratives.

For many countries and regions outside of the West, there is limited information on the prevalence of Long COVID and post-COVID illness. The reason for this lack of information varies between regions. Some nations, particularly those in East and Southeast Asia, suppressed transmission of the virus through strict social precautions in the early pandemic, meaning that post-COVID illness may be less common in these parts of the world when compared to the West. However, in other parts of the world with limited healthcare resources, it is unclear whether a lack of data on post-COVID illness reflects a lower prevalence of illness, or whether the post-COVID disability that does exist is not being recorded or linked to COVID. An important consideration is that chronic health issues that may be considered uncommon or exceptional in the West—such as malaria, tuberculosis, anemia, and general ill health and infections from malnutrition or poor sanitation—are commonplace in poorer parts of the developing world. In this type of environment, COVID's acute flu-like symptoms and variable long-term health effects could be lost in the noise of other common illnesses that produce similar symptoms. Although data on Long COVID's global prevalence is incomplete, the global spread of COVID-19 means that nearly every country on Earth will have at least some people who experience lasting health complications from COVID-19 infection. Future action on Long COVID should acknowledge it as a global health issue and incorporate perspectives on chronic illness from outside of just a Western medical perspective.

3.1 Europe

Western Europe was the first epicenter of COVID-19 to emerge outside of China in early 2020, and the 44 countries of the European continent have continued to experience multiple waves and high case numbers throughout 2021 and 2022. Patterns in pandemic activity in Europe, such as the spread of new variants, are generally mirrored in the US with a short delay due to the high rates of air travel and connectedness between these two regions. Typically regarded as wealthy, industrialized countries with strong universal healthcare systems, the shocks caused by the early waves of COVID-19 greatly overwhelmed the healthcare capacity of Western European nations.

The horrors of the first COVID-19 wave recorded in wealthy and well-resourced parts of Europe, such as Italy's Lombardy region, amplified the fear of what the pandemic could mean for countries in the Global South with larger populations, under-resourced healthcare systems, and limited access to advanced medical care. European survivors of the early COVID-19 waves played an important role in organizing the first Long COVID patient groups and patient-led studies into the condition—eventually leading to medical recognition of the phenomenon in the summer of 2020 (Callard and Perego 2021).

As the pandemic has progressed into 2021 and 2022, and COVID-19 vaccines have become available, Europe has adopted a heavily vaccine-focused response to COVID-19 with little appetite for lockdowns, movement restrictions, and other social interventions since the initial lockdowns of early 2020. Such interventions have raised concerns about civil liberties within political blocs such as the European Union, which guarantees freedom of movement between citizens of member states, as well as fears of harsh economic fallout. As a result of such attitudes, recent surges in COVID-19 cases (i.e., Omicron) saw the return of only a few social restrictions in Europe. Instead, the response of most countries in the winter of 2021–2022 relied on high vaccine coverage and efficacy to prevent surges in severe illness, hospitalization, and death (Onishi and Casey 2021).

Within this vaccine and severe illness-focused COVID-19 response framework, Long COVID has occupied little space in the official European narrative. The disease has been acknowledged by the health systems of Western European countries with high infection rates, such as the UK, France, Germany, and Spain, with modest amounts of funding being allocated toward research and the operation of post-COVID clinics. In many European countries, post-COVID clinics and healthcare services are targeted toward individuals who were hospitalized with severe illness, and the demand for these services far outweighs the available capacity. Except for in the UK (discussed in the next section), there has been relatively little surveillance of post-COVID illness within the general, non-hospitalized population, and patients around Europe are calling on their governments for more action on Long COVID (Baraniuk 2022).

While European Long COVID patients are experiencing long wait times and few options beyond supportive and specialist-based care at government-run post-COVID clinics, some European countries have become medical tourism destinations for people seeking experimental Long COVID treatments. These treatments, which are run out of private clinics in countries such as Germany, Sweden, and Cyprus, operate based on informed consent models in which patients willingly accept the risks and costs of these treatments. These treatments occupy a complex space within the post-COVID environment, and their existence can be seen as an indictment of the failure of "gold-standard" scientific protocols to adequately address the urgency of the Long COVID health crisis.

3.1.1   The UK

The UK's Office of National Statistics (ONS) estimated in May 2022 that two million people in the UK, or approximately 3% of the population, were living with long-term illness from COVID-19. Of the responses obtained from this national survey, 70% of people reporting Long COVID symptoms reported a negative impact on their daily lives, and 20% reported severe impairment (Davis 2022). In some regards, the UK has emerged as a global leader in Long COVID surveillance within their general population and the establishment of a network of post-COVID clinics—capabilities that are facilitated by strong centralized data collection from institutions such as the National Health Service (NHS) and ONS. However, it could also be argued that the UK is a global leader in addressing Long COVID because the bar for this title is painfully low—any effort to address Long COVID as a real health issue looks admirable when compared to limited, slow-moving, or nonexistent actions being taken by most governments globally.

Indeed, the UK's Long COVID response itself is one born out of necessity. A February 2022 report by the ONS estimated that 70% of people in the UK had been infected with COVID-19 between the start of the pandemic and the winter 2021–2022 Omicron surge (Devlin 2022). This infection rate—one of the highest in the world—is the result of policy decisions that promoted mass infection with the end goal of achieving natural herd immunity (Thomson 2021). This goal failed due to the lack of long-term immunity provided by wild-type COVID infection and vaccination against immune-evasive mutated strains such as the Delta and Omicron variants, resulting in recent waves of repeat and breakthrough infections. This failed gamble for herd immunity also resulted in a wave of long-term disability among COVID survivors that threatened to swamp the NHS— and more noticeably—exacerbated labor shortages (Reuschke and Houston 2022). The population-level impact of Long COVID resulting from mass infection became too large to ignore.

In response to the demand for post-COVID medical care, the NHS established a post-COVID plan in June of 2021 that outlined ten next steps for the advancement of post-COVID care in the UK (NHS 2021). The steps included £100 million allocated to the expansion of post-COVID clinics and primary care services, better care coordination, establishment of pediatric care centers, expansion of a digital post-COVID rehabilitation platform, and more data collection. These steps and allocations are meant to expand the reach of the NHS's post-COVID clinics, of which over 80 have been set up across the UK (primarily in England—fewer services are available in Scotland, Wales, and Northern Ireland).

NHS post-COVID clinics are run by multidisciplinary teams and essentially serve as triage centers for Long COVID patients who were previously hospitalized or who have been referred to the clinic through primary care. Patients referred to these clinics undergo batteries of tests to assess which of the many possible Long COVID symptoms they are most affected by and are provided with a treatment plan based on these assessments. The screening process utilized by these clinics sorts symptoms into three management levels (See Fig. 3.1):

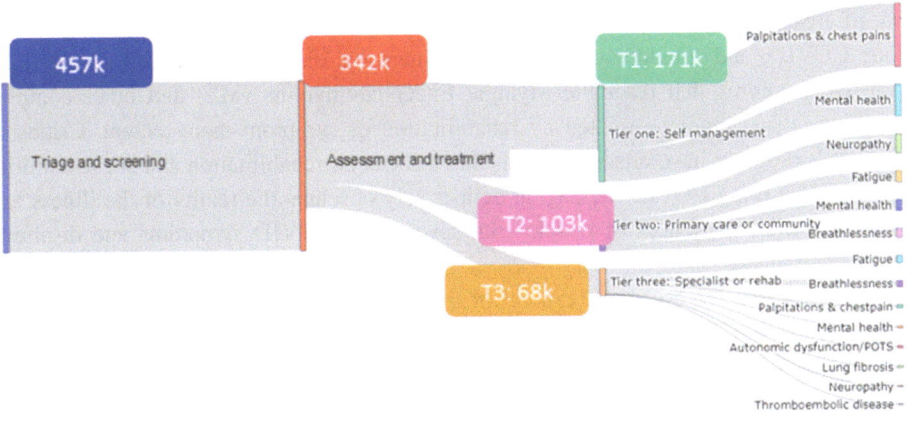

Fig. 3.1 NHS's indicative flow of patients with long COVID symptoms (NHS 2021)

- **Tier 1**: Self-management of symptoms such as palpitations, chest pain, and mild mental health issues. Management of these symptoms is done at home using tools such as the NHS's "Your COVID Recovery" app. NHS reports place 30–50% of post-COVID patients in this category.
- **Tier 2**: Primary or community-based care for symptoms such as neuropathy, milder fatigue, moderate mental health issues, and breathlessness. These patients may be referred back to their general practitioner/primary care provider with a treatment plan. The NHS places 18–30% of patients in this category.
- **Tier 3**: Specialist care or rehab for a range of post-COVID symptoms that necessitate this level of care. For these patients (20–50%), the post-COVID clinic provides a referral to a specialist or rehabilitation service for a specific symptom.

Long COVID patients have been critical of the NHS's program. Some patients have found the centers to be helpful resources—reporting symptom relief from their treatment plan or having found the acknowledgment of the illness itself by a medical authority to be helpful. However, other patients see the current approach as insufficient in addressing their symptoms and the burden of Long COVID as a whole. Perhaps the most obvious criticism of the NHS's Long COVID program is its inability to absorb the full extent of the demand for post-COVID medical care in the UK. Given the ONS's estimate of two million people in the UK living with Long COVID symptoms, expecting the existing post-COVID clinic system to handle this problem at scale is an impossible ask, even if the system's capacity was expanded beyond the existing 80–90 clinics. With the mismatch between the capacity and demand for post-COVID care and downstream specialty care services, patients often wait months for appointments that provide underwhelming treatment or relief for their agonizing symptoms.

The other main criticism leveraged against the UK's post-COVID clinic system is that its treatment approach does nothing to address the underlying biological causes of Long COVID, and provides only a few treatment options to people with severe Long COVID symptoms that resemble Myalgic Encephalomyelitis (ME) and other complex conditions that cannot be treated by rehabilitation or symptom management. Critics of the NHS's program have raised concerns that a focus on rehabilitation and success stories in the NHS's Long COVID messaging deliberately obscures the reality of the illness and minimizes the experiences of people with severe post-COVID symptoms and disability (The Telegraph 2021).

ME advocates are especially critical of the NHS's program due to the Graded Exercise Therapy (GET)/Cognitive Behavioral Therapy (CBT) controversy—a recent fight over the guidelines that outline best care practices for ME, and by extension, Long COVID. Up until their revision in October 2021 (NICE 2021), the UK NICE guidelines for ME recommended GET as a treatment for ME, despite any form of physical activity being contraindicated for Post-Exertional Malaise (PEM)—the hallmark symptom of ME in which physical or mental exertion causes energy crashes and permanently decreased function. The guidelines also recommended CBT for patients with ME—a therapy that patient advocates saw as promoting the harmful idea that ME is a psychological illness instead of a severe form of physiological dysfunction (Friedberg 2016). Despite the updated guidance, the biopsychological model of ME and other IACIs such as Long COVID remains pervasive, and patient advocates have raised the alarm about the risks that rehabilitation-based treatment plans pose for Long COVID patients with comorbid ME.

3.1.2 Continental Europe and Medical Tourism

People experiencing post-COVID symptoms in Western countries that have experienced high numbers of COVID cases may come into contact with the healthcare system in a variety of ways. Most hard-hit European countries, such as Belgium, France, Germany, and Spain, have established post-COVID specialist clinics in some capacity. However, the reach of these clinics in continental Europe lags behind the NHS post-COVID clinic system seen in the UK, with most of these resources being targeted at post-hospital patients (Baraniuk 2022). Similar to the situation in the UK, these European post-COVID clinics have limited capacity and primarily serve as triage centers. After testing and assessment at a clinic, patients are often referred back to primary care to develop an individualized treatment plan with their doctor. The clinics themselves, in the meantime, continue to triage and refer patients outside their clinic to work through their long waitlists.

Patients who are triaged through post-COVID clinic systems in Europe, the UK, and the US have expressed intense frustration with the inability of their countries' healthcare systems—which are often touted as some of the most advanced in the world—to provide answers or relief to their debilitating symptoms. Many patients perceive medical practitioners as dismissive of their suffering—by attributing intractable symptoms to psychological illness instead of working to find, or even admitting that they do not know the underlying physiological cause. The psychologizing dismissal of Long COVID can occur in multiple places within the triage system. Some patients may be referred to mental health practitioners after their clinic assessment, while others may never be able to get in the door if their primary care provider attributes their Long COVID symptoms to anxiety and refuses to give them a clinic referral.

Despite the long backlogs and inefficiency of the official, state-sanctioned European post-COVID systems, some European countries, such as Germany, Austria, Sweden, and Cyprus, have become medical tourism destinations for long-haulers who can afford the costs of travel and private treatment. The services and treatments that are offered by private clinics around Europe vary widely—practices range from promising-but-invasive biomedical procedures, to off-label use of existing drugs, to scientifically questionable wellness procedures and drug therapies that have previously been touted for acute COVID or a wide swath of other health concerns. These experimental treatment clinics operate under an informed consent model that is allowed under European laws, permitting doctors to prescribe off-label medicine. However, the costs of private treatment can be high, and clinics may operate under ethically dubious practices that have raised concern about the financial, legal, and physical risks that individuals are taking to relieve their Long COVID symptoms.

The most positively touted form of experimental Long COVID treatment within patient groups is Heparin-induced Extracorporeal LDL Precipitation (HELP) apheresis, a blood-filtering procedure that is based on the hypothesis that microscopic blood clots (microclots) contribute to a significant portion of Long COVID symptoms. This procedure is based on research by Dr. Resia Pretorius and her colleagues, which identified abnormal clotting and amyloid-based microclots in patients with Long COVID (Pretorius et al. 2021). This hypothesis is built on pre-existing research on abnormal clotting and vascular damage as a mechanism for respiratory and organ failure during acute COVID infection (Ackermann et al. 2020; Iba et al. 2020), as well as evidence of respiratory hypoperfusion (reduced blood flow to the lungs) in Long COVID patients (Buonsenso et al. 2021).

The microclot theory hypothesizes that these clots, which are often too small to be detected by standard tests, may induce systemic ischemia and hypoxia by blocking blood flow in capillaries—leading to organ damage, fatigue, cognitive dysfunction, and low oxygen extraction (Singh et al. 2021). The treatment that is being used to remove microclots from the blood is known as HELP apheresis, a dialysis-like procedure in which a heparin filter removes unwanted lipids and proteins from the blood before returning it to the patient's body (Davies 2022). Anecdotal reports of rapid symptom alleviation following apheresis treatment indicate a relationship between the clotting pathology and Long COVID symptoms that treatment proponents want to see followed up with larger-scale research.

Experimental treatments—even ones that hold promise for future research and treatment—are not without their risks. The lack of regulation over off-label and experimental treatments exacerbates many of these risks and creates a landscape in which the legitimacy and safety of a treatment varies between privately-run clinics. For example, private Long COVID clinics that focus on clotting pathologies often prescribe multiple anticoagulant drugs to patients undergoing treatment. Patients who are prescribed anticoagulant drugs typically must undergo routine medical supervision due to the increased risk of severe bleeding from these treatments and the narrow therapeutic index (NTI) of drugs such as Warfarin that necessitate highly specific dosing and frequent prescription adjustments (Eikelboom and Hirsh 2006; U.S. Food and Drug Administration 2022). The lack of appropriate surveillance and follow-up with these types of treatments poses risks for patients undergoing unregulated treatments—especially if they are traveling abroad to do so.

Additionally, experimental Long COVID treatments may be sold to consumers at high prices or in conjunction with scientifically dubious treatments such as dietary supplements, off-label hyperbaric oxygen therapy, and debunked COVID-19 "treatments" such as hydroxychloroquine (Stephens 2022). The out-of-pocket costs for experimental Long COVID treatments and the travel needed to undergo them mean that these interventions are accessible only to the wealthy—or to people who are desperate enough to drain their life savings (Tait 2022).

Long COVID patients who are undergoing assessment through post-COVID programs cannot be referred to experimental private clinics because state- and institutionally-run programs are unwilling to assume the same risks that some individuals are choosing to undertake. The lack of gold-standard clinical approval for biomedical Long COVID treatments, such as large-scale clinical trials, is often cited by post-COVID programs and practitioners as the reason for refusing to recommend these treatments. From a regulator's standpoint, promising experimental treatments are just as unproven and risky as alternative medicine "miracle cures", if there is insufficient data to show the effectiveness of treatment beyond a small experimental population.

These regulators argue that without clinical trials and established standards of care, bringing experimental treatments into the fray of Long COVID care introduces an unacceptable level of risk to patients. Proponents of experimental treatments, on the other hand, believe that this adherence to slow-moving, "business-as-usual" scientific protocols drastically underestimates the risk that postponing or withholding Long COVID treatment poses to patients (Davies 2022). How much more risk can experimental treatments pose to patients who are already suffering from severe untreatable illness, burning through their life savings, and becoming homeless due to the current status-quo approach?

Biomedical treatment proponents are also quick to point out that for all the skepticism leveled at experimental therapies such as HELP apheresis due to a lack of clinical trials, there has been little movement on the part of institutions such as the National Institutes of Health (NIH) and NHS to provide the funding that would allow these clinical trials to take place (Putrino 2022). Much of the diagnostic- and treatment-based Long COVID research that has been performed has taken place outside of the traditional funding apparatus, through private funding and even crowdfunded campaigns (Kernls 2022).

The current showdown between state-run and private approaches to Long COVID care and treatment in Western countries demonstrates a vacuum of authority on Long COVID, as the medical system's inability to provide patients with little more than symptom management has left many patients feeling ignored and desperate. Patients who are experiencing severe and poorly understood illness are being forced to either wait indefinitely for validated research and treatments, or to seek relief in a web of unregulated treatments that run the gamut from promising biomedical interventions to snake oil treatments that can cure everything from Long COVID to autism to cancer (depending on who you ask!). In attempting to protect patients from risky and unproven treatments, advocates of the scientific status quo have ironically worsened the very problem they were trying to avoid.

Medicine's failure to help desperate Long COVID patients has increased their distrust in the medical system and made them more amenable to alternative medicine, medical tourism, and other practices that medical authorities try to discourage. However, given Western medicine's long history of neglect toward chronic, complex, and post-infection illness, resorting to such measures can be seen as a rational response on the part of patients—just one that brings a large amount of individual risk with it. Incidences of Long COVID-related medical tourism may become more frequent and occur in more parts of the world if the availability of treatments that alleviate patient concerns continues to be an issue.

3.2   Latin America

The story of the spread of COVID-19 and attempts to control it in Latin America can be seen as both tragic and underwhelming. Throughout the pandemic, Latin America has experienced a consistent spread of COVID-19, without the large surges experienced in Europe and North America, but without breaks in transmission either. Most Latin American countries (except Brazil, a notable outlier which is discussed below) initially enacted a strict COVID lockdown response which sharply constrained movement and economic activity. These lockdowns were implemented before the virus reached Latin America and were lifted when the virus was beginning to spread. The containment measures, despite being early, were ill-timed to contain the virus and inflicted a significant economic wound on the region, with the International Monetary Fund (IMF) estimating a 7.4% economic contraction for the region in 2020 (Werner et al. 2021). The limited effectiveness of lockdown measures and economic relief efforts is attributed to high regional rates of informal employment.

An estimated 30% of people in Latin America make a living through precarious in-person work and small businesses that are not registered with the state. People who rely on this type of work for their income were unable to stay home or stop working—resulting in low adherence to lockdown measures—while at the same time being ineligible for state-sponsored economic relief programs (Knowles and Healey 2022). The low institutional capacity of bureaucratic governments in Latin America to implement effective relief programs is blamed for the failure of these interventions—an institutional flaw that some economists blame for the existence of Latin America's large informal economy in the first place (De Soto 1989).

Across much of Latin America, the economic turmoil and social inequality exacerbated by the pandemic and the political elite's ineffective response to long-standing social issues have been a larger story than the virus itself. Mass protests were seen in countries such as Columbia, Peru, Ecuador, and Chile against human rights violations, inequality, political repression, and food and fuel shortages—often being met with brutal police crackdowns (Rojas 2021). Public discontent with governments led to regime shifts in Columbia and Bolivia, and a re-writing of Chile's constitution that prioritizes social equality and human rights (Barry 2022). Amid this political backdrop, COVID-19 has received more attention as an example of institutional failure and a reason for public discontent than as a story by itself.

The most glaring example of failed government responses to COVID-19 in Latin America is that of Brazil's far-right president Jair Bolsonaro—a failure in leadership that resulted in so many deaths that some Brazilian senators want it investigated as a crime against humanity (Downie 2022). Brazil is by far the Latin American country most heavily infected by COVID-19, with over 33 million cases and 600,000 deaths—the second highest death rate in the world behind the US (WHO 2022). Brazil's public health system, which had successfully handled recent disease outbreaks such as H1N1 influenza in 2009 and Zika in 2015, was weakened throughout the Bolsonaro administration by budget cuts and political appointments of military personnel with no public health background.

Once COVID-19 began spreading in Brazil, Bolsonaro refused to lock down the country, publicly dismissed the threat posed by the virus, and rallied against protective measures such as face masks and vaccines while promoting conspiracy theories and false COVID cures. The lack of federal response to COVID-19 caused the Brazilian public health response to be coordinated almost entirely at the state and local level. The backlash against Bolsonaro's extreme COVID-denialist policies led to the establishment of local vaccination campaigns that have helped mitigate the pandemic and contribute to high vaccination rates in some parts of the country.

An early 2021 study of the impact of COVID-19 on the Brazilian healthcare system warned of a "third wave" of the pandemic characterized by an influx of patients with worsened chronic illness. This warning was made not in reference to Long COVID, but instead to the delays in screenings, diagnoses, and routine care for people living with noncommunicable illnesses (Bigoni et al. 2022). The strain that Long COVID is likely to exert on Latin American healthcare systems, especially in Brazil due to its exceptionally high infection rate, adds to the existing concern about the system's capacity to absorb excess long-term illness.

Given the political situation surrounding acute COVID in Latin America, it is no surprise that governments in this region have paid little attention to Long COVID and taken no steps to collect data or address it at a systemic level. Most of the attention on Long COVID in Latin America comes from researchers in countries such as Brazil and Mexico who are seeking to characterize the illness through cohort studies. These studies have found a high prevalence of Long COVID symptoms in sample cohorts (50–68%), although these rates may be attributable to most studies focusing on survivors who visited emergency rooms or were hospitalized (De Miranda et al. 2022; Wong-Chew et al. 2022). Other studies have focused on characterizing the range of symptoms experienced by Long COVID patients rather than identifying the prevalence of the illness (Bonifacio et al. 2022).

Of the studies published in Latin America so far, there is a strong focus on neurological and psychiatric symptoms being among the most common and distressing sequelae (Flores-Silva et al. 2021). In one study of a Mexican post-hospital cohort, seven of the ten most common lingering symptoms (fatigue, headache, sadness, alopecia, insomnia, desire to cry, anguish, anger, anhedonia, and back pain) (Wong-Chew et al. 2022) fell under the neuropsychiatric umbrella. Concerns about the neuropsychiatric and mental health impacts of Long COVID are not unique to Latin America—studies out of Africa and India also draw particular attention to these symptoms.

However, legitimate concern about the mental health impact of Long COVID and the trauma of the pandemic is a complex topic, since attributing Long COVID symptoms to mental health conditions such as anxiety is often used to dismiss physical symptoms and deny specialist referral (France 24 2021b). Focus on Long COVID as an illness with primarily neuropsychiatric manifestations could be an opportunity to pay more attention to the impact of COVID-19 on the brain, or to justify the medical neglect of patients that healthcare systems are not set up to handle.

3.3 Asia

The Asian continent, which contains 60% of the world's population and its two most populous countries, has had a range of experiences with COVID-19 across its many regions. Most Asian countries enacted a stronger COVID response than the West during 2020, using their centralized (and in some cases, authoritarian) governments to enact strict lockdowns, segregate infected individuals into quarantine centers, mandate testing and masking across the population, and provide infected individuals with food and other necessary supplies enabling them to isolate and avoid moving through public spaces. Through these measures, much of the Asian continent was able to control cases and avoid surges in 2020 and early 2021. However, these strict infection control measures had harsh economic consequences and struggled to suppress more contagious and immune-evasive variants.

In regions such as the Middle East and South Asia, migrant laborers were a particularly vulnerable group that bore the brunt of the initial lockdowns while having limited access to healthcare and economic prospects. Meanwhile, in East and Southeast Asia, the impacts of pandemic lockdowns on the manufacturing and tourism industries placed an unsustainable burden on many countries' economies. Most Asian countries have experienced surges in COVID-19 as of 2022, with the protections of most countries failing in the winter of 2021–2022 due to the hyper-contagious Omicron variant and the opening of borders to international travelers. China—the last holdout with its "Zero COVID" policy—abruptly dropped its protections at the end of 2022 and experienced a predictably massive surge in cases. The long-term impacts of this surge, which impacted 18% of the global population in the span of a month, will likely never be fully known or publicized.

Although most Asian countries have experienced low rates of COVID-19 infection until recently, one major country stands out as the most heavily affected by COVID and Long COVID—India.

3.3.1 India

In the Spring of 2021, as COVID-19 case numbers plummeted in Western countries due to the rollout of the COVID-19 vaccines, a horror story was brewing in India and other parts of South Asia. A hyper-contagious variant of COVID-19, which would come to be known as the Delta variant, had evolved and was spreading like wildfire through India's population. India, the second most populous country on Earth, had enforced a strict lockdown for its population of 1.3 billion people in the early waves of COVID-19. This approach helped slow the spread of the virus but created a humanitarian crisis for the country's estimated 140 million migrant workers. These workers, many of whom were employed in low-wage manual labor and service jobs in cities hundreds of miles from their home villages, suddenly found themselves stranded and cut off from any means of employment and income. With the country's lockdown blocking access to public transportation such as trains, these workers were left with little choice but to walk back to their home villages. Efforts to provide these workers with food, shelter, and economic support failed due to local food shortages and the failure of biometric authentication technologies, as well as a lack of participation by some local governments (Shaji 2020). A survey of 11,000 Indian migrant workers found that 96% did not receive government rations, and 90% were not paid by their employers during the lockdown (The Hindu 2020).

By early 2021, cases were on the decline in India as the country rolled out its vaccination program and earlier pandemic restrictions and emergency infrastructure were being dismantled. The rapid emergence and spread of the Delta variant, which caused more severe illness than previous strains of COVID-19 in addition to being more transmissible, caught India's population off-guard. The rapid spread off the illness is attributed to multiple factors, including the variant itself, the return of young people into social life, weddings, and large festivals, and pressure to reopen to relieve the harsh economic impact of earlier lockdowns (Hindustan Times 2021; Indian Express 2021). At the peak of the Delta wave, India was reporting over 400,000 cases of COVID-19 a day, with many additional cases going untested and unreported. The rapid rise of COVID-19 cases overwhelmed hospitals and created a critical shortage of supplemental oxygen—leading to mass death among patients whose lives could have been saved if oxygen had been available. In July 2022, India reported 44 million COVID-19 cases and over 500,000 deaths—the second highest cumulative number of cases in the world after the US (Ritchie et al. 2022).

India's catastrophic experience with the Delta variant resulted in a radical shift in the country's management of the virus—one that has maintained strong measures to prevent the country from being caught off guard by a new COVID variant again. At the core of India's COVID response is substantial investment into COVID surveillance technologies such as PCR testing and genome surveillance to identify emerging variants. All positive COVID test samples collected at India's state-run testing sites are sequenced to identify the variant responsible for the infection—a policy that allows outbreaks and new variants to be identified and contained early (Raina 2023). The Indian government's messaging on the pandemic has emphasized the importance of continuing to take precautions against COVID. In contrast to many Western countries, India has not treated regional downturns in positive cases as an end to the pandemic as a whole, and remains vigilant of the virus's continued mutation and spread in other parts of the world (Raina 2023).

The Indian government's continued surveillance of COVID-19 in the country has allowed preventative measures, such as mask mandates, quarantines, and screening of travelers, to be applied and relaxed regionally in response to the virus's activity and emerging outbreaks. In addition to these measures being mandated by state and local governments during outbreaks, many Indians also continue to voluntarily take individual-level precautions such as masking (Dayal 2022). Compliance with precautionary measures such as quarantines is assisted by government-sponsored aid programs, which provide food rations and other resources that enable people who test positive for the virus to stay home and not move around their community while infectious (Raina 2023).

While vaccine resistance is an issue in some rural communities, largely fueled by online and peer-to-peer misinformation, these views are uncommon—an estimated 2–3% of Indians have refused the COVID vaccine, compared to 19% of Americans (Changoiwala 2022). The majority of Indians, by contrast, have received at least one COVID vaccine dose. As a result of the Indian government's COVID policies that were adopted in response to the Delta wave in 2021, and the willingness of most citizens to comply with government guidelines, India has maintained low COVID-19 transmission and avoided additional large national outbreaks throughout 2022 and 2023.

India's experience with widespread COVID infection in 2020 and 2021 has created a cohort of people within the country who have developed additional health problems and long-term illness following infection (Naik et al. 2021; Anjana et al. 2021). The Indian Ministry of Health and Family Welfare (IMHFW) released guidelines for treating post-COVID illness in 2020, after the people infected in the first wave of the pandemic began developing health complications. Post-COVID illness is acknowledged by Indian healthcare authorities and providers, but with a different approach than the concept of Long COVID originating in the West. Instead of being grouped together under a post-COVID label, patients with new post-COVID health issues, such as heart problems, diabetes, or neurological issues, are absorbed into the healthcare system as patients of that particular illness type. For example, a patient who develops cardiac issues post-COVID is treated as a regular cardiac patient. The IMHFW's guidelines on the management of post-COVID illness highlight the 5 medical specialties observing the highest influx of patients with post-COVID sequelae: cardiology (heart), gastroenterology (GI tract), nephrology (kidneys), neurology (brain, as well as fatigue and dysautonomia), and pulmonology (respiratory system) (IMHFW 2023).

Hospital systems and NGOs in India have also set up post-COVID clinics for patients with more complex, multisystemic forms of illness—those who fall more under the label of 'Long COVID'. These clinics take a multidisciplinary approach to diagnosis and treatment, and can offer patients customized care and rehabilitation plans. These specialized clinics were established by some Indian hospital systems as early as 2020—meaning that even prior to the surge in cases from the Delta variant, Indian doctors and scientists were aware of the potential for long-term illness, and had observed that some patients infected during the first wave failed to recover (Dasgupta 2020). The IMHFW has continued to take post-COVID illness seriously into the present, through policies such as establishing more post-COVID clinics across the country, directing money into research on post-COVID health issues, and establishing post-COVID cardiac clinics in all medical colleges (The Hindu 2023).

While Indian healthcare providers—particularly specialists—have reported increased patient loads and younger patients being seen for specialty care post-COVID, this influx has been largely absorbed by the private side of India's healthcare system (Raina 2023). Compared to many Western hospital systems that are struggling due to staff shortages, Indian healthcare has more staff and greater slack built into the system. This feature of the system was designed to accommodate the common occurrences of seasonal illness in India, which routinely stretch the healthcare system beyond its usual operating capacity. While India's public clinics and healthcare facilities have fewer resources than private facilities (Kapasi 2022), other recently-enacted public health policies have worked to take some of the strain off of this part of the healthcare system. These policies include a public health insurance program (Ayushman Bharat) that covers general and specialist care for the poorest half of India's population (INHA 2019), and rules allowing patients to access specialist care within the private healthcare system without a referral from a general practitioner—hence freeing up space within the public system (Raina 2023). Finally, India's ongoing COVID mitigation policies have helped limit patients with post-COVID disabilities to a defined cohort, instead of a constant influx of patients disabled from new waves of the virus.

India continues to face a range of public health concerns from both infectious and chronic forms of illness, particularly among its poorest residents. The health complications caused by COVID-19 add another layer on top of this existing disease burden. However, India's response to the pandemic—which has emphasized acknowledgement of the risks posed by COVID-19; continued surveillance and communication surrounding the virus; and investments in healthcare infrastructure—has reduced the spread of the virus without imposing prolonged lockdown or invasive mitigation measures. Some elements of India's COVID response are examples of realistic policies that other governments could take to mitigate the ongoing pandemic. However, others represent more significant long-term investments in healthcare and social infrastructure that will require time, money, and political willpower for other countries to be able to replicate.

3.4   Africa

The outcomes of the COVID-19 pandemic have upended previous assumptions about global health preparedness and which countries are the best and worst equipped to deal with a pandemic. Wealthy Western countries, which are typically considered to have advanced healthcare systems, have struggled to control COVID-19 and its aftereffects due to weak political will to contain the virus. On the other hand, regions of the world such as sub-Saharan Africa, which many experts feared would be defenseless in the face of COVID-19, have seen less disease burden from COVID-19 than anticipated. Sub-Saharan Africa is in the midst of the epidemiological transition, in which the bulk of disease burden shifts from infectious diseases to non-communicable diseases (NCDs), such as heart disease, cancer, and diabetes. This trajectory of development has been nonlinear due to HIV and co-occurring infectious diseases such as tuberculosis causing a regression in population health during the 1990s and 2000s (Kabudula et al. 2017).

While access to antiretroviral treatment (ART) has reversed this trend by making HIV a manageable illness, this condition remains one of many chronic conditions that leaves people vulnerable to infectious diseases. An "unprecedented" rise in the rates of NCDs in sub-Saharan Africa, and interactions between these illnesses and HIV/AIDS, was being reported before the emergence of COVID-19 (National Research Council 2012). COVID-19 has elicited concerns because it is an airborne "equal-opportunity" disease, in contrast to other infectious diseases in Africa that cause more severe illness, but are generally concentrated to specific regions or groups (Knowles and Steere-Williams 2021).

As one of parts of the world where infectious disease outbreaks are a recent and extant threat (WHO 2020a, b, c, d, e, f), governments in sub-Saharan Africa were determined to keep COVID-19 out of their countries in the early pandemic, knowing that the level of mass illness seen in other parts of the world would rapidly collapse their healthcare systems. African governments also knew that once COVID-19 vaccines and therapeutics were developed, their access to them would depend on foreign donations and that supply would be limited. COVID-19 outbreaks also threatened to exacerbate and undo progress on other public health initiatives, such as childhood vaccination programs, malnutrition, and access to essential healthcare services (WHO 2020a, b, c, d, e, f).

These known challenges that would arise if COVID-19 became widespread in Africa led most governments to adopt a strict and cautious approach to COVID-19 that lasted well into 2021 (WHO 2020a, b, c, d, e, f). Containment measures in the early pandemic included police- and military-enforced lockdowns, restrictions on internal travel, border closures, suspension of international air travel, prohibition of mass gatherings, and nightly curfews in urban areas (Knowles 2021; Haider et al. 2020). These restrictions were eventually loosened or lifted due to their harsh economic impact—particularly on impoverished people relying on public transportation and in-person work for survival (WHO 2020a, b, c, d, e, f).

Much of the public health focus on COVID-19 in Africa has centered around vaccination and the myriad challenges in ensuring adequate vaccine coverage across Africa. Despite Africa lagging behind many other parts of the world in vaccine coverage, with 20% of the population being fully vaccinated as of July 2022 (Africa CDC 2022), the continent has seen much lower rates of death from COVID-19 than wealthy Western countries. This trend is believed to be due to multiple factors, including early containment-focused policies and Africa's young population that is at reduced risk from severe illness and death from COVID-19 (France 24 2021a). A late 2020 report by the WHO found that 91% of COVID-19 infections in sub-Saharan Africa were in people under the age of 60 (WHO 2020a, b, c, d, e, f). However, the picture of the COVID infection rate in Africa is murky—this same report found that 80% of infections in their sample were asymptomatic, meaning that a significant number of COVID cases in Africa may go completely unreported.

Testing capacity in most sub-Saharan African countries is well below that of European countries, and seroprevalence samples in countries such as Kenya, Malawi, and Mozambique have found COVID-19 antibodies in a larger percentage of the population than the low reported case numbers would suggest (Nordling 2020). South Africa—the most heavily affected country in Africa according to official case counts—has reported case and death rates over ten times higher than other sub-Saharan African countries, and accounts for one-third of the official cases. However, it is unclear to what extent these statistics represent true differences in infection rates, considering that South Africa has the testing infrastructure to run nearly ten times the number of COVID tests per capita compared to other African nations (Haider et al. 2020).

Long COVID has received little to no attention from African governments or media, and Long COVID cases are addressed by medical systems on a case-to-case basis. The lack of data and surveillance of COVID cases in Africa—particularly the mild and asymptomatic cases that make up most of the infections on the continent—makes it difficult to determine the disease burden posed by Long COVID. The problem certainly is not non-existent—South African doctors have spoken out about how Long COVID has been seen in Africa since 2020, but a majority of the focus has been on the much more pressing acute illness. Doctors who are seeing Long COVID patients in South Africa report that 10–20% of survivors report ongoing symptoms, with medical pathologies being found in 40% of the survivors.

Special concern has been raised about the ongoing neurological effects of Long COVID, and the high rates of depression and mental health issues being seen in patients (Newzroom Afrika 2022; WHO 2020a, b, c, d, e, f). Long COVID also poses an elevated risk for people living with HIV, which affects over 15% of the population in South Africa and neighboring southern African countries. Although COVID-19 poses the greatest risk of death to people who are seriously immunocompromised from HIV infection, people living with ART-controlled HIV are still four times more likely to develop Long COVID than people without HIV (Alcorn 2022). The rise in NCDs triggered by COVID-19 infection is likely to exacerbate pre-pandemic concerns about rising NCD rates and the ability of African healthcare systems to adequately care for them. The complex systemic disease seen in some Long COVID cases will be a step beyond that.

For all the challenges that Long COVID poses to African healthcare infrastructure, social structures based in community solidarity and support may provide a buffer against the worst social outcomes for people living with Long COVID in Africa. These norms, such as the door-to-door vaccination work of community health workers and the pooling of community resources, helped mitigate the worst effects of COVID-19 within some communities. One cultural tradition, described by Kenyan writer and political analyst Nanjala Nyabola, is the Kenyan cultural ethos of generosity known as *Harambee* (Musau 2020), in which community members rally around and pool resources to help a community member who is undergoing a form of hardship such as severe illness (Knowles 2021).

These community-level norms and safety-net structures exist in response to a long history of government neglect and a lack of public expectation of government assistance for community-based crisis responses. During the pandemic, these community pools were used to support people who were facing exorbitant medical bills after hospitalization. Such a form of community support resembles the phenomenon of online medical crowdfunding, which many COVID long-haulers have been forced to rely on for survival. Although people in this example from Africa receive multiple types of support (i.e., food, interpersonal, in-kind) from family and community members, instead of monetary donations from online acquaintances or generous strangers, both strategies portend the forms of support that long-haulers around the world may come to rely on for their continued survival.

3.5   Discussion

Long COVID has received a relatively small amount of attention on the global stage, when compared to the public health issues that characterized the acute stage of the pandemic—such as death rates, hospitalizations, and vaccination. As the acute stage of the pandemic transitions towards a more 'endemic' stage—in which COVID continues to spread and mutate without causing the massive surges seen early in the pandemic, we can expect to inhabit a world with higher rates of post-COVID disability. At this inflection point of the pandemic, how countries choose to address and prepare for this ongoing public health crisis will have important geopolitical ramifications. Acknowledging the long-term impacts of COVID, and investing in the healthcare, research, and social support systems needed to mitigate these effects, will prove to be a geopolitical asset in the coming decades—especially for countries who are already rising in prominence on the world stage. Conversely, refusal to address the effects of COVID-19 beyond the acute illness stage will diminish countries' abilities to respond to a world that is becoming increasingly defined by complexity and crisis.

The global response to Long COVID has been slow, in part, because of the lack of diagnostics and treatments that have undergone enough scientific and regulatory scrutiny to be used in an organized fashion. Although research into the biological underpinnings of Long COVID has uncovered promising biomarkers, clinical tools are still in their experimental phase. Individuals with the means to travel and pay out-of-pocket for private treatments have been able to access to these treatments.

However, state- and institutionally-run clinics are unable and unwilling to refer patients for experimental treatments, and generally offer little more to patients than tools for symptom management. This conflict is a major source of frustration for Long COVID patients, who feel that the health crisis posed by Long COVID is too great and urgent to wait for the years-long clinical trial process. The lack of funding for biomedical Long COVID research that would enable these clinical trials has raised further concern about near-future treatment prospects as the number of Long COVID cases continues to rise.

Given that COVID-19 has spread to nearly every country on Earth, Long COVID can be expected to become a global health issue that intersects with other ongoing health and social crises that existed before the pandemic. However, much of the existing attention on Long COVID has been focused on high-income Western countries, such as the US, Canada, the UK, and European countries. This pattern reflects both historical patterns of health and medical research being concentrated in high-income countries and the higher COVID infection rates in these parts of the world. Low- and middle-income countries, except for hard-hit nations such as India and Brazil, have seen little government or institutional acknowledgment of Long COVID.

Western treatment models may not be feasible for some low- and middle-income countries if the battery of diagnostic tests used in Long COVID assessment is unaffordable to patients. However, the failure of the Western medical model to adequately research and treat Long COVID draws the assumed superiority of this model into question. IACIs, such as ME, are a long-running exception to Western medicine's proclaimed ability to treat severe illness, and the number of people that are falling through the cracks because of this failure raises concerns about Western countries' ability to lead research on this emerging global health issue. Will countries in other parts of the world with sufficient research bases be able to pick up the slack?

In many of the countries that have acknowledged Long COVID, the focus of research and treatment has been on formerly hospitalized patients. This approach does make sense, given that both acute and Long COVID have been handled using a triage model throughout the pandemic. People hospitalized for COVID also exhibit higher rates of lingering COVID symptoms and disabilities acquired during hospitalization, such as Post-Intensive Care Syndrome (PICS), Post-Traumatic Stress Disorder (PTSD), deconditioning, and cognitive decline. However, this focus omits the fact that most people with Long COVID were never hospitalized, and that mild and asymptomatic cases of COVID can lead to debilitating Long COVID symptoms.

This has created an informational gap among medical professionals treating Long COVID patients that has had to be filled by patients themselves. Only a minority of Long COVID patients have been able to take on the role of patient advocates and activists—doing so typically requires technological literacy, internet access, connection to communities of people with similar symptoms, and the social capital to refute people in positions of medical authority. Long COVID patients around the world who lack these privileges face the greatest risk of harm from the medical community's lack of comprehensive education on Long COVID. Awareness of COVID's impact on a wide range of body systems and disease processes on the part of medical providers—thereby reducing the onus on patients to self-advocate—can help mitigate this harm.

Research on Long COVID symptoms around the world has found roughly the same commonly reported symptoms, such as fatigue, muscle pain, shortness of breath, and cognitive dysfunction, across cohorts. One interesting trend is that Long COVID studies out of the Global South, such as Latin America, India, and Africa, have focused on neurological and psychiatric symptoms as particularly common and concerning. Neuropsychiatric symptoms of concern include mood disturbances (i.e., depression, apathy, agitation), anxiety, brain fog, forgetfulness—and perhaps drawing the most concern—severe sleep disturbances.

These neuropsychiatric characterizations of Long COVID exist within a complicated and fraught diagnostic space. Long COVID symptoms such as heart palpitations caused by orthostatic intolerance can be easily misdiagnosed as anxiety, and psychiatric diagnoses are commonly used to dismiss intractable physical symptoms caused by chronic illness. At the same time, COVID-19 has known impacts on the brain, and many Long COVID patients worldwide have experienced serious trauma and life stress from the pandemic—which they are forced to deal with on top of their newly developed illness.

The current global response to Long COVID is piecemeal—not only is supportive care distributed on an individual level, but each country is also being left to coordinate its own response with little overarching guidance. The absence of coordinated leadership on this issue has resulted in a reactive response to Long COVID in many countries. Countries are only motivated to establish post-COVID clinics when the volume of Long COVID patients becomes so large that it is impossible to ignore—such as when patients begin to overwhelm primary and specialist care, or when this illness has a noticeable impact on the workforce.

The reactive response to Long COVID continues into the clinic, where symptoms of complex illness are treated separately by practitioners operating within their silos of expertise. Long COVID is an example of a healthcare crisis that governments and healthcare systems around the world are not well-set up to address. The lack of action on Long COVID threatens the health and well-being of millions of people around the world and threatens the public health progress that many countries have worked so hard to achieve.

References

Ackermann M, Verleden S, Keuhnel M (2020) Pulmonary vascular endothelialitis, thrombosis, and angiogenesis in COVID-19. N Engl J Med 2020; 383:120–128. https://doi.org/10.1056/NEJMoa 2015432

Africa CDC (2022) COVID-19 vaccine dashboard. Africa CDC. https://africacdc.org/covid-19-vac cination/. Accessed 20 Sept 2022

Alcorn K (2022) Long COVID more common in people with HIV. Aidsmap. https://www.aidsmap. com/news/mar-2022/long-covid-more-common-people-hiv. Accessed 20 Sept 2022

Anjana N, Annie T, Siba S et al (2021) Manifestations and risk factors of post COVID syndrome among COVID-19 patients presented with minimal symptoms—A study from Kerala, India. Journal of Family Medicine and Primary Care. https://doi.org/10.4103/jfmpc.jfmpc_851_21

Baraniuk C (2022) COVID-19: How Europe is approaching long COVID. BMJ. https://doi.org/10. 1136/bmj.o158

Barry E (2022) Chile is trying to shed the last remnants of its pinochet-era dictatorship. Time. https:// time.com/6193719/chile-constitution-reform-boric/. Accessed 20 Sept 2022

Bigoni A, Malik AM, Tasca R et al (2022) Brazil's health system functionality amidst of the COVID-19 pandemic: An analysis of resilience. The Lancet Regional Health. https://doi.org/10.1016/j. lana.2022.100222

Bonifacio L, Csizmar V, Barbosa-Junior F (2022) Long-term symptoms among COVID-19 survivors in prospective cohort study, Brazil. Emerg Infect Dis. 28:730–733. https://doi.org/10.3201/eid 2803.212020

Buonsenso D, Di Giuda D, Sigfrid L et al (2021) Evidence of lung perfusion defects and ongoing inflammation in an adolescent with post-acute sequelae of SARS-CoV-2 infection. The Lancet Child & Adolescent Health. https://doi.org/10.1016/S2352-4642(21)00196-6

Callard F, Perego E (2021) How and why patients made long COVID. Soc Sci Med. https://doi.org/ 10.1016/j.socscimed.2020.113426

Changoiwala P (2022) In Rural India, Extreme Covid Vaccine Hesitancy. Undark. https://undark. org/2022/04/26/in-rural-india-extreme-covid-vaccine-hesitancy/. Accessed May 25, 2023.

Dasgupta D (2020) Dedicated clinics in India provide specialised care to 'long Covid' patients. The Straits Times. https://www.straitstimes.com/asia/south-asia/dedicated-clinics-in-india-pro vide-specialised-care-to-long-covid-patients. Accessed May 27, 2023.

Davies M (2022) Long COVID patients travel abroad for expensive and experimental blood washing. BMJ 2022; 378. https://doi.org/10.1136/bmj.o1671

Davis N (2022) Two million people in UK living with long COVID, find studies. The Guardian. https://www.theguardian.com/world/2022/jun/01/two-million-people-in-uk-living-with-long-covid-say-studies. Accessed 20 Sept 2022

Dayal S (2022) India on lookout for new COVID variants as cases in other countries climb. Reuters. https://www.reuters.com/world/india/india-step-up-covid-surveillance-cases-increase-elsewh ere-2022-12-21/

De Miranda D, Gomes S, Filgueiras P (2022) Long COVID-19 syndrome: A 14-months longitudinal study during the two first epidemic peaks in southeast Brazil. Transactions of The Royal Society of Tropical Medicine and Hygiene. https://doi.org/10.1093/trstmh/trac030

De Soto H (1989) The other path. New York, New York: Harper & Row Publishers, Inc.

Devlin H (2022) Seven in 10 people in England have had COVID, research shows. The Guardian. https://www.theguardian.com/world/2022/apr/22/seven-in-10-people-in-england-have-had-covid-research-shows-omicron. Accessed 20 Sept 2022

Downie A (2022) Outrage in Brazil as jair bolsonaro avoids five charges related to COVID response. The Guardian. https://www.theguardian.com/world/2022/jul/27/outrage-brazil-jair-bolsonaro-avoids-five-charges-related-to-covid-response. Accessed 20 Sept 2022

Eikelboom J, Hirsh J (2006) Monitoring unfractionated heparin with the APTT: time for a fresh look. Thromb Haemost. 96:547–52. https://pubmed.ncbi.nlm.nih.gov/17080209/. Accessed 20 Jan 2022

Flores-Silva FD, Garcia-Grimshaw M, Valdes-Ferrer SI et al (2021) Neurologic manifestations in hospitalized patients with COVID-19 in Mexico City. PLOS One. https://doi.org/10.1371/journal.pone.0247433

France 24 (2021a) Africa records surge in COVID-19 cases, but fewer deaths than before, says WHO. France 24. https://www.france24.com/en/africa/20211214-africa-records-surge-in-COVID-19-cases-but-fewer-deaths-than-before-says-who. Accessed 20 Jan 2022

France 24 (2021b) Mexico's overstretched doctors face another foe: long COVID. France 24. https://www.france24.com/en/live-news/20210227-mexico-s-overstretched-doctors-face-another-foe-long-covid. Accessed 20 Jan 2022

Friedberg F (2016) Cognitive-behavior therapy: why is it so vilified in the chronic fatigue syndrome community? Fatigue: Biomedicine, Health & Behavior. https://doi.org/10.1080/21641846.2016.1200884

Haider N, Osman AY, Gadzekpo A (2020) Lockdown measures in response to COVID-19 in nine sub-Saharan African countries. BMJ Global Health 2020;5:e003319. https://doi.org/10.1136/bmjgh-2020-003319

Hindustan Times (2021) Superspreader events like weddings behind new COVID surge: Govt panel. Hindustan Times. https://www.hindustantimes.com/india-news/superspreader-events-like-weddings-behind-new-covid-surge-govt-panel-101616177606318.html. Accessed 20 Jan 2022

Iba T, Levy J, Levi M, Thachil J (2020) Coagulopathy in COVID-19. J Thromb Haemost. 18:2103–2109. https://doi.org/10.1111/jth.14975

IMHFW (2023) National Comprehensive Guidelines for Management of Post-COVID Sequelae. Indian Ministry of Health and Family Welfare. https://www.mohfw.gov.in/pdf/NationalComprehensiveGuidelinesforManagementofPostCovidSequelae.pdf

Indian Express (2021) Despite surge in cases, COVID guidelines flouted during Holi celebrations. Indian Express. https://indianexpress.com/photos/india-news/covid-19-holi-celebrations-7250394/7/. Accessed 20 Jan 2022

INHA (2019). About Pradhan Mantri Jan Arogya Yojana (PM-JAY). Indian National Health Authority. https://nha.gov.in/PM-JAY.html. Retrieved 28 May 2023.

Kabudula C, Houle B, Collinson M (2017) Progression of the epidemiological transition in a rural South African setting: findings from population surveillance in Agincourt, 1993–2013. BMC Public Health. https://bmcpublichealth.biomedcentral.com/articles/10.1186/s12889-017-4312-x. Accessed 20 Jan 2022

Kapasi S (2022) Personal Communication. June 19, 2022.

Kernls (2022) Develop an accessible, lab-based method to diagnose microclots in long COVID patients. https://kernls.com/projects/diagnose-longcovid-microclots. Accessed 20 Sept 2022

Knowles SG (2021) History and Politics of Public Health Intervention in Kenya. [Audio Podcast Episode]. COVID Calls #367

Knowles SG, Healey M (2022) Disasters and COVID in latin america w/ Mark Healey [Audio Podcast Episode]. COVID Calls #461. https://www.youtube.com/watch?v=ifm_6xiarla. Accessed 20 Sept 2022

Knowles SG, Steere-Williams J (2021) South Africa, HIV/AIDS, and epidemiology w/ Guest Host Jacob Steere-Williams [Audio Podcast Episode]. COVID Calls #319.

Musau MM (2020) Harambee: The law of generosity that rules Kenya. BBC. https://www.bbc.com/travel/article/20201004-harambee-the-kenyan-word-that-birthed-a-nation. Accessed 20 Jan 2022

Naik S, Haldar S, Soneja M et al (2021) Post COVID-19 sequelae: A prospective observational study from Northern India. Drug Discoveries & Theraputics. https://doi.org/10.5582/ddt.2021.01093

National Research Council (US) (2012) The Continuing epidemiological transition in sub-saharan Africa: A workshop summary. Washington (DC): National Academies Press (US); 2012. 8, The Epidemiological Transition in Africa: Are There Lessons from Asia? Available from: https://www.ncbi.nlm.nih.gov/books/nbk114529/

Newzroom Afrika (2022) Is South Africa approaching long COVID and its effects adequately? https://www.youtube.com/watch?v=hqs3nuihmyy. Accessed 20 Sept 2022

NHS (2021) Long COVID: The NHS plan for 2021/22. National Health Service England. https://www.england.nhs.uk/coronavirus/documents/long-covid-the-nhs-plan-for-2021-22/. Accessed 20 Sept 2022

NICE (2021) NICE ME/CFS guideline outlines steps for better diagnosis and management. National Institute for Health and Care Excellence. https://www.nice.org.uk/news/article/nice-me-cfs-guideline-outlines-steps-for-better-diagnosis-and-management. Accessed 20 Jan 2022

Nordling L (2020) The pandemic appears to have spared Africa so far. Scientists are struggling to explain why. Science. https://www.science.org/content/article/pandemic-appears-have-spared-africa-so-far-scientists-are-struggling-explain-why. Accessed 20 Jan 2022

Onishi N, Casey N (2021) Crack down hard, or wait and see? Europe splits on omicron response. New York Times. https://www.nytimes.com/2021/12/20/world/europe/europe-divided-omicron-response.html. Accessed 20 Jan 2022

Pretorius E, Vlok M, Bezuidenhout J et al (2021) Persistent clotting protein pathology in long COVID/post-acute sequelae of COVID-19 (PASC) is accompanied by increased levels of antiplasmin. Cardiovascular Diabetology. https://doi.org/10.1186/s12933-021-01359-7

Putrino D [@PutrinoLab] (2022, July 15). After 8 months, we just received the news that @NIH will not be funding our #long COVID microclot study. They declined to provide reviewer comments. I'm so sorry to everyone in the community who was counting on this work, I don't know what to say other than we will keep fighting [Tweet]. https://twitter.com/PutrinoLab/status/1547978525331693571. Accessed 20 Sept 2022

Raina S (2023) Personal Communication. May 23, 2023.

Reuschke D, Houston D (2022) The impact of long COVID on the UK workforce. Applied Economics Letters. https://doi.org/10.1080/13504851.2022.2098239

Ritchie H, Mathieu E, Rodes-Guirao (2022) Coronavirus pandemic (COVID-19). Our World in Data. https://ourworldindata.org/coronavirus

Rojas N (2021) Protests, inequality, and brutal crackdowns in Latin America. The Harvard Gazette. https://news.harvard.edu/gazette/story/2021/11/harvard-panel-discusses-protests-across-latin-america/. Accessed 20 Jan 2022

Shaji L (2020) Flattening the curve at the expense of one's constitutional rights? Centre for Constitutional Research and Development. https://ccrd.vidhiaagaz.com/migrant-workers-flattening-the-curve-constitutional-rights/. Accessed 20 Jan 2022

Singh I, Joseph P, Heerdt P et al (2021) Persistent exertional intolerance after COVID-19. Chest 161:54–63. https://doi.org/10.1016/j.chest.2021.08.010

Stephens M (2022) Desperate Americans are going abroad for unproven long COVID cures. The Daily Beast. https://www.thedailybeast.com/long-covid-sends-desperate-americans-abroad-for-cures. Accessed 20 Jan 2022

Tait A (2022) COVID clinics: hope and high prices on the long road to recovery. The Guardian. https://www.theguardian.com/global/2022/jan/02/covid-clinics-hope-and-high-prices-on-the-long-road-to-recovery. Accessed 20 Sept 2022

The Hindu (2020) 96% migrant workers did not get rations from the government, 90% did not receive wages during lockdown: survey. The Hindu. https://www.thehindu.com/data/data-96-migrant-workers-did-not-get-rations-from-the-government-90-did-not-receive-wages-during-loc kdown-survey/article31384413.ece. Accessed 20 Jan 2022

The Hindu (2023) More post-COVID-19 clinics being set up in all districts: Minister. The Hindu. https://www.thehindu.com/news/national/kerala/more-post-covid-19-clinics-being-set-up-in-all-districts-minister/article66563687.ece. Accessed May 27, 2023

The Telegraph (2021) What happens at a long COVID clinic as 1m people in the UK have long-term symptoms? [Video Communication]. https://www.youtube.com/watch?v=fpcm9xhhkpq. Accessed 20 Jan 2022

Thomson H (2021) Herd immunity to COVID-19 may not be attainable in the UK. New Sci. 251(3348):17. https://doi.org/10.1016/S0262-4079(21)01448-2

U.S. Food and Drug Administration (2022) Warfarin INR test meters. https://www.fda.gov/medical-devices/in-vitro-diagnostics/warfarin-inr-test-meters. Accessed 20 Sept 2022

Werner A, Ivanova A, Komatsuzaki T (2021) Latin America and Caribbean's winding road to recovery. International Monetary Fund. https://blogs.imf.org/2021/02/08/latin-america-and-car ibbeans-winding-road-to-recovery/. Accessed 20 Jan 2022

WHO (2020a) 24 September 2020a WHO regional office for Africa. https://whotogo-whoafrocc master.newsweaver.com/journalenglishnewsletter/12oe7dsqud4y48iiujdam4?lang=en&a=2&p= 57860491&t=31103707. Accessed 20 Jan 2022

WHO (2020b) COVID-19 could deepen food insecurity, malnutrition in Africa. WHO Regional Office for Africa. https://whotogo-whoafroccmaster.newsweaver.com/journalenglishnewsletter/ ara078231nty48iiujdam4?email=true&lang=en&a=11&p=57028129. Accessed 20 Jan 2022

WHO (2020c) COVID-19 halting crucial mental health services in Africa, WHO survey. WHO Regional Office for Africa. https://whotogo-whoafroccmaster.newsweaver.com/journalenglishn ewsletter/469cokb2ijky48iiujdam4?email=true&lang=en&a=11&p=57959447. Accessed 20 Jan 2022

WHO (2020d) COVID-19 hits life-saving health services in Africa. WHO Regional Office for Africa. https://whotogo-whoafroccmaster.newsweaver.com/journalenglishnewsletter/1l8t7w ec3zvy48iiujdam4?email=true&lang=en&a=11&p=58142773. Accessed 20 Jan 2022

WHO (2020e) COVID-19 pandemic expands reach in Africa. WHO Regional Office for Africa. https://whotogo-whoafroccmaster.newsweaver.com/journalenglishnewsletter/jo9xudvqxuoy48i iujdam4?email=true&lang=en&a=11&p=568143500. Accessed 20 Jan 2022

WHO (2020f) The African region reinforces preparedness for coronavirus disease. WHO Regional Office for Africa. https://whotogo-whoafroccmaster.newsweaver.com/journalenglishnewsletter/ 62uxehwl61ay48iiujdam4?email=true&a=11&p=56444925. Accessed 20 Jan 2022

WHO (2021) A clinical case definition of post COVID-19 condition by a Delphi consensus, 6 October 2021. https://www.who.int/publications/i/item/who-2019-ncov-post_covid-19_condition-cli nical_case_definition-2021.1. Accessed 20 Jan 2022

WHO (2022) COVID 19 dashboard—Brazil. World Health Organization. https://covid19.who.int/ region/amro/country/br. Accessed 20 Sept 2022

Wong-Chew RM, Rodriguez Cabrere EX, Rodriguez Valdez CA et al (2022) Symptom cluster analysis of long COVID-19 in patients discharged from the Temporary COVID-19 Hospital in Mexico City. Therapeutic Advances in Infectious Disease. https://doi.org/10.1177/20499361211069264

COVID-19 Versus Past Pandemics: What Can We Learn?

4

COVID-19 may be a novel virus, but the social and political dynamics linked to it are not unique. This chapter explores several historical and modern pandemics that each provide new understandings of the COVID-19 pandemic and its aftermath:

- The first outbreak examined is the 2003 Severe Acute Respiratory Syndrome (SARS) epidemic, caused by SARS-COV, a genetic relative of the SARS-COV-2 virus.
- The second is a set of three pandemics that occurred in the late nineteenth and early twentieth centuries: the 1918 Influenza Pandemic, the 1915–1926 Encephalitis Lethargica Pandemic, and the 1889–1890 Russian Flu. These three related pandemics are the closest modern analog to the scale of the COVID-19 pandemic and provide insight into the political aftermath of a mass casualty and mass-disabling event.
- Human Immunodeficiency Virus (HIV)/AIDS and its establishment of the modern patient activist movement is explored as a precursor to mobilization around ME/CFS and Long COVID.

4.1 Severe Acute Respiratory Syndrome (SARS)

The first modern disease outbreak that may provide insight into the long-term trajectory of people with Long COVID and other COVID-19 sequelae is the 2003 SARS outbreak. The SARS-COV virus originates from the same coronavirus family as SARS-COV-2, and the two viruses are genetically similar (Abdelrahman et al. 2020). Both viruses target ACE2

© The Author(s), under exclusive license to Springer Nature Switzerland AG 2024
M. Smallwood, *The Future of Long COVID*, Synthesis Lectures on Threatcasting,
https://doi.org/10.1007/978-3-031-40474-0_4

(Li et al. 2003)—an inflammation-modulating cell receptor found throughout the body—and produce similar respiratory symptoms during acute infection. However, despite the similarities between these two related viruses, the trajectory of their spread around the world is very different. Some of these differences are due to the unique disease characteristics itself, but many are attributable to the behavioral and organizational responses to these outbreaks.

The SARS outbreak began in China's Guangdong Province in November 2002, and most the global cases associated with the outbreak occurred between February and July of 2003. Approximately 8,000 cases were recorded globally throughout the outbreak—the majority of which occurred in China, Taiwan, Hong Kong, and other East Asian countries. Outside of East Asia, the largest outbreak of approximately 250 cases occurred in Toronto, Canada. Of the 8,000 recorded cases, 800 deaths were recorded, indicating a case fatality ratio of 10 percent that far exceeds the mortality rate of COVID-19.

When compared to SARS-COV-2, the SARS-COV virus tended to create more severe acute disease and a lower incidence of asymptomatic cases. This facet of the disease, combined with a shorter incubation period and lower transmissibility (compared to SARS-COV-2), allowed most cases of the disease to be identified and quarantined before SARS could spread substantially across the globe (Wilder-Smith et al. 2020).

SARS was contained before becoming a true global pandemic due to a strong, top-down public health response in affected countries. SARS was the first major respiratory disease outbreak to occur in a modern, globalized context. Air travel was identified as the source of rapid spread between continents, with travel advisories being created and publicized over major news networks in response. The context in which SARS emerged was an important component in the willingness of people in affected communities to voluntarily comply with public health measures such as testing, symptom surveillance, and community quarantines.

The public health response that averted the development of the SARS outbreak into a global pandemic resulted in this disease incident having relatively little long-term societal or cultural impact outside of East Asia. However, longitudinal studies following the small cohort of people who survived SARS have found that a significant percentage of survivors experienced serious long-term disability from their infections. One 2004 rehabilitation program studied the impairments experienced by 50 Canadian healthcare workers who had been infected with SARS—one-fifth of the total Canadian SARS outbreak (Patcai 2022).

The study found multiple lingering effects of infection, including (1) low blood oxygen saturation and gas exchange (despite normal lung function), (2) limited capacity for physical activity, (3) multiple neurological, psychiatric, and cognitive issues, and most significantly, (4) severely disturbed sleep patterns. Within this 50-person sample, no participants reported being able to work at their pre-infection capacity—some were completely unable to work, while others tried and failed to return to their previous job positions and daily activities. Most continued to rely on caretakers for activities of daily living, and none reported a return to their pre-infection normal.

Other meta-analyses of post-SARS literature have found significant rates of disability among SARS survivors. A meta-analysis by Chau et al. (2021) found mental health complications in 20–30% of SARS survivors across studies (Chau et al. 2021). However, this meta-analysis focused only on the common psychiatric diagnoses of depression, anxiety, and PTSD—it did not examine the wider array of neuropsychiatric and sleep-related issues found in the Canadian study. A four-year post infection follow-up study by Lam et al. (2009) found that within a sample of 369 SARS survivors in Hong Kong, 40% reported ongoing psychiatric illnesses and 27% met the criteria for ME/CFS. Additional studies have found elevated rates of pulmonary fibrosis and bone necrosis among SARS survivors, years after infection (Zhang et al. 2020).

Until a resurgence of interest in the disease in 2020 due to the COVID-19 pandemic, SARS had a relatively low impact on society outside of the small, unfortunate cohort of people whose bodies and minds were ravaged by this disease. However, as COVID-19 continues to spread across the globe, leaving large numbers of people with similarly severe medical complications in its wake, new attention should be paid to what we know about the long-term trajectory of SARS and its relatives. Specifically, the fact that the most persistent SARS sequelae are not the respiratory symptoms that characterize acute COVID-19, but the more pervasive and complex neurological issues, should raise the alarm that the healthcare challenges posed by Long COVID are not the same as the ones prioritized for acute COVID.

4.2 Spanish Flu, Russian Flu and Encephalitis Lethargica: Pandemics in the Age of Eugenics

4.2.1 Influenza Pandemic of 1918

The Influenza Pandemic of 1918—commonly referred to as the "Spanish Flu"—is the best-known pandemic in recent history and the one that is most frequently used as a point of comparison for COVID-19 due to its global scale. The 1918 pandemic occurred in three waves between 1918 and 1919, and is estimated to have infected over 500 million people—or one-third of the total global population—and resulted in over 50 million deaths. The novel strain of influenza (H1N1) that caused the 1918 pandemic was exceptional for its high rate of mortality in young people—particularly those regarded as robust and healthy.

Typical seasonal influenza is known for its elevated risk of death for the very young and very old, while posing a relatively small risk of severe disease for adults under the age of 65. However, the opposite pattern of mortality was seen in the 1918 pandemic—a pattern that is believed to be caused by an out-of-control immune response (cytokine storm) triggered by this strain of the virus (Short et al. 2018). The strong immune response that would normally protect young adults from severe disease may have instead contributed to the high rate of death, with the body's attempts at targeting the virus causing widespread tissue damage and leaving the patient susceptible to fatal pneumonia and opportunistic bacterial infections.

The social and political context of the 1918 pandemic is inseparable from World War I (WWI) (Crosby 2003). The origin of the pandemic is believed to be a Kansas military base. Although it is disputed (and likely never to be known) whether the virus originated there or if the military base's cramped conditions simply provided it with ideal conditions for rapid spread, it is undoubtable that the mass movement of American military troops across the Atlantic into Europe in the final year of WWI caused the initial spread of the 1918 influenza virus across the world. Like the role that airplane travel plays in the global spread of modern respiratory illnesses, the ships that transported troops around the world spread the virus within military garrisons and port cities across continents, which seeded simultaneous civilian outbreaks in far-flung parts of the globe.

The 1918 pandemic was not recognized as a disease of concern in the US by the civilian population and newly established public health services until the second wave of autumn 1918, which was the deadliest wave of the pandemic. Even while military and civilian healthcare systems alike were overwhelmed with an influx of patients suffering from pneumonia and other severe flu complications, the outbreaks were overshadowed by the political situation surrounding the war effort. In some cases, outbreaks were attributed to a wartime German plot to weaken the US and similar political conspiracies. Mass gatherings inspired by the war effort, such as Philadelphia's ill-fated Liberty Loan Parade in September 1918, resulted in super-spreading and large outbreaks. However, most people of the time did not seek medical care until their illness necessitated it and carried on with their everyday lives if their illness remained mild. Soldiers with the flu particularly avoided military hospitals due to their overcrowded conditions, inexperienced staff, and the fear of being permanently separated from their company.

Although the pandemic of 1918 is known to be the twentieth century's largest mass disease event, specific records and statistics about the multitude of outbreaks that occurred around the world are often incomplete and spotty. Many of the most reliable records about the outbreaks in the US originate from military organizations—both because of the impact of the virus on troop readiness and the surveillance and monitoring systems put in place by these organizations. Civilian cases, on the other hand, were not reliably reported until the height of the second wave in the autumn of 1918, as the virus was not regarded as a reportable disease until then. Even after pandemic influenza was labeled as a reportable illness, overwhelmed doctors and hospitals often failed to report cases on top of their other duties, and there was little to no disease reporting in the rural Western states. Estimates of the total cases were often extrapolations of retroactive surveys and canvasses, and the most reliable metric of the scope of the 1918 pandemic is its mortality rate.

The 1918 pandemic is known for its high rate of acute illness and death, and few records exist regarding the sequelae and long-term effects of pandemic influenza. Ill health and early death were not uncommon or unusual in the early twentieth century. Common infectious diseases that have since been eradicated from the developed world were commonplace, and medical science had not yet developed effective treatments, cures, or basic scientific understanding of most ailments. However, a lack of record-keeping on this subject does not mean that the 1918 pandemic did not incur significant health consequences. Longitudinal and census-based cohort studies of children born during the 1918 pandemic have found their exposure to the H1N1 influenza virus in utero was correlated with lower educational accomplishments, higher rates of illness and disability later in life, lower socioeconomic status, and increased reliance on social services (Almond 2006).

Additionally, high-profile cases of people experiencing health decline and illness following an influenza infection did exist—including the president of the US Woodrow Wilson. President Wilson became seriously ill with the flu in April 1919 during the Paris Peace Conference. During the course of his illness, Wilson was bedridden, fatigued, and experienced unpredictable behavioral changes and delusions. After his initial illness, those close to the President reported that he never regained his former strength or mental acuity, that he had difficulty making simple decisions, and that he continued to experience paranoid and odd beliefs. President Wilson suffered a severe stroke in October of 1919, which left him incapacitated until his death in 1924 (Solly 2020).

4.2.2   Encephalitis Lethargica

The Encephalitis Lethargica pandemic is a lesser-known outbreak of neurological illness that took place in the shadow of the active havoc of the 1918 Influenza pandemic. This outbreak is believed to have affected over one million people between the years of 1915 and 1926, with over 500,000 deaths, and to this day, is still considered a medical mystery. Encephalitis Lethargica was believed to be caused by a viral infection of the brain that led to severe neurological sequelae, such as Parkinsonian symptoms, catatonia, lethargy, and an inability to direct attention. As described by neurologist Oliver Sacks in his book *Awakenings* (Sacks 1999).

> They would be conscious and aware – yet not fully awake; they would sit motionless and speechless all day in their chairs, totally lacking energy, impetus, initiative, motive, appetite, affect or desire; they registered what went on about them without active attention, and with profound indifference. They neither conveyed nor felt the feeling of life; they were as insubstantial as ghosts, and as passive as zombies.

Encephalitis Lethargica patients who did not recover on their own had little hope for treatment or a return to a normal life. Most were institutionalized and slowly deteriorated or died over the decades. *Awakenings* tells the story of the discovery of L-dopa as a treatment for Encephalitis Lethargica patients. Although the miraculous recovery of the patients in this story shed newfound light on the cause and treatment of this devastating illness, this intervention came decades too late for most people who had become disabled in the 1910s and 1920s. Even the patients who recovered thanks to L-dopa lost over four decades of their lives to illness.

The severe disturbances in consciousness, sleep, and movement that occurred in patients with Encephalitis Lethargica are believed to have been caused by an out-of-control autoimmune reaction in the midbrain and basal ganglia (Dale et al. 2004). However, the infectious agent responsible for this condition is less certain. The largest and last known outbreak of Encephalitis Lethargica overlapped with the 1918 pandemic, but it is disputed whether the H1N1 influenza virus directly caused these severe neurological sequelae, or if it simply rendered people and populations more vulnerable to other viral infections. Other infectious agents that have been implicated in Encephalitis Lethargica are Staphylococcus bacteria (BBC 2004) and the virus responsible for the 1889–1890 pandemic known as the "Russian Flu".

4.2.3 "Russian Flu" of 1889

The Pandemic of 1889–1890, also known as the Russian Flu, was one of the deadliest pandemics in history—killing over 1 million people out of a 1.5 billion global population. For most of the twentieth century, the 1889 pandemic was believed to be an influenza pandemic due to its primary symptoms being respiratory, febrile, and flu-like in nature. However, during the 2003 SARS outbreak, a re-examination of historical data spawned an alternate theory—that the infectious agent responsible for the Russian Flu was a coronavirus. Interest in this theory has understandably increased during the COVID-19 pandemic, with particular attention being paid to the high rate of long-term neurological sequelae reported in survivors of the 1889 pandemic.

When historical accounts of the 1889 pandemic are compared to contemporary outbreaks of SARS and COVID-19, the disease's symptoms and attack pattern appear to resemble coronavirus infections more so than common influenza or even the super-virulent H1N1 influenza that caused the 1918 pandemic. The moniker "Russian Flu" is a colloquial name given to the illness based on its respiratory systems—scientific understanding of viruses did not exist until the 1930s. The acute symptoms of the 1889 virus are described as coughing, fever, chills, body pain, fatigue, rashes, and skin abnormalities on the extremities.

These symptoms displayed a rapid onset, and many patients experienced a false recovery period in which they briefly recovered from their initial symptoms only to suffer a more severe secondary relapse (Vijgen et al. 2005). Other aspects of the virus's behavior that more closely resemble coronaviruses than influenza are (1) evidence of asymptomatic and pre-symptomatic transmission, (2) elevated risk of mortality in the elderly, (3) exacerbation of underlying comorbidities, (4) the presence of variable long-term sequelae in approximately 10% of survivors, and perhaps most interestingly—(5) the loss of taste and smell that is currently recognized as a unique indicator of COVID-19 infection (Brussow and Brussow 2021).

Historical accounts of the 1889 pandemic report a range of symptoms in survivors that strongly resemble post-SARS and post-COVID sequelae and indicate damage and dysregulation of multiple organ systems. These symptoms include long-term physical and mental weakness, dizziness and vertigo, cardiac symptoms, and "cardiac depression with general arterial relaxation necessitating recourse to the recumbent position" (Vijgen et al. 2005)—that would today be recognized as dysautonomia or POTS, neurological symptoms, and multi-system organ damage. Other historical accounts report symptoms across the cardiac, respiratory, gastrointestinal, dermatological, and neurological systems (Kousoulis and Tsoucalas 2017).

Long-term neurological sequelae, such as depression, anxiety, fatigue, and an inability to concentrate attention stand out in historical reports as the longest lasting sequelae of the 1889 pandemic—a pattern that is also observed in post-SARS, post-COVID, and Encephalitis Lethargica patients. Cases of Encephalitis Lethargica—colloquially referred as "Nona"—were recorded as a "mystery illness" during the 1889 pandemic in parts of Europe such as Italy and Hungary (JAMA 1919). With regard to Long COVID, it is important to note that neurological symptoms and multi-organ damage are the most significant sequelae of these past pandemics—not the respiratory symptoms that define the acute stages of these illnesses.

4.2.4   Pandemics and the Road to Fascism

The three pandemics of the late nineteenth and early twentieth centuries discussed above took place in the decades prior to one of the most violent and politically unstable periods of the modern era—World War II and the global spread of fascism. The political extremism, hyper-nationalism, and global conflict of the 1930s and 1940s arose from a complex array of socioeconomic and geopolitical factors, and no single factor can be "blamed" for the conflicts and atrocities of this era.

However, the contemporary American political landscape has seen nationalist and far-right ideology gain a foothold and move into mainstream political conversation since the early 2010s through movements such as the Tea Party, and more recently, the rhetoric of former President Donald Trump. The pandemic has rapidly accelerated these political trends through the politicization and violent opposition toward efforts to mitigate the spread of COVID-19, such as vaccination, masking, and school closures. The prospect of widespread disability becoming evident in the years following the highly politicized

COVID-19 pandemic has raised alarms due to the role that ideas surrounding disability, weakness, and dependency have played in historical fascist and far-right movements.

Historical accounts of pandemics tend to focus on death rates, with comparatively little coverage of the long-term health impacts of these diseases on survivors. There are multiple reasons for this trend; deaths are easy to understand and measure and are limited to a specific point in time, versus disability, which is often subjective and requires measurement over months or years. The stress that disease outbreaks place on societies favors action and surveillance against acute illness, hospitalization, and death, with long-term disability being an after-thought or not a factor to begin with. However, there may also be a darker and more worrying reason for the erasure of post-infection disability from records of the late nineteenth and early twentieth century pandemics: the eugenics movement.

The eugenics movement began in the 1880s and dominated much of Western science and medicine until the 1940s—only publically falling out of favor once the atrocities of the Holocaust and Nazi extermination programs based around this ideology were exposed to the world. Prior to World War II, eugenics was viewed as a tool to improve the human race through selective breeding and the elimination of "undesirable" traits. Informed by the "race science" of the nineteenth century, eugenics categorized people with Northern and Western European ancestry as genetically superior to people of other races, and was used as a justification for colonialism, segregation, and involuntary sterilization of racial minorities.

Additionally, the eugenics movement regarded social issues like poverty, crime, and various forms of disability (i.e., "feeblemindedness") as the products of poor genetics, with little regard for environmental and social factors. The sterilization and institutionalization programs that ensued from this ideology were openly touted as a public good by early twentieth century medical and public health authorities (Rivard 2014). Eugenic attitudes toward disability and social issues pushed by medical authorities were met with widespread cultural valorization of masculinity and strength (often tied to patriotic or nationalistic sentiment) and a hatred of weakness, vulnerability, and femininity. This ideology would go on to inspire some of the worst atrocities of the twentieth century.

In his 1995 essay *Ur-Fascism* (Eco 1995), Italian historian Umberto Eco describes fourteen features that define fascist ideology. Eco describes fascism as a "cult of traditionalism" that cultivates unquestioning faith and loyalty to the State and its all-powerful leader and a reactionary hatred for any form of weakness, dissent, or outside influence that "threatens" this vision. Fascist ideology views the State as a sort of organism unto itself, in which individual identity and agency is subsumed for the good of the whole. As an extension of this "organism" metaphor, undesirable aspects of society are frequently framed in terms of disease and disability (e.g., a minority group being compared to a diseased organ or limb that must be removed). However, a closer examination of the role that both disease and its metaphors play in fascist rhetoric reveals a much more complex and twisted relationship between the two.

Fascists hold two seemingly contradictory beliefs regarding infectious disease. Right-wing authoritarian leaders (and their followers) who were in power during the COVID-19 pandemic—such as the US' President Donald Trump, Brazil's Jair Bolsonaro, and Russia's Vladimir Putin—were notorious for mocking and disregarding evidence-based medical and public health measures to reduce the spread of COVID-19. Supporters of these leaders mocked and violently protested non-pharmaceutical interventions such as masking and quarantines. Anti-vaccine conspiracy theories also flourished with the tacit or open approval of right-wing leaders. From the beginning of the pandemic, right-wing followers seemingly went out of their way to catch and spread COVID-19 far and wide.

However, while right-wing ideology mocks public health interventions to control the spread of disease, ideas about sickness, disability, and contamination also have an obsessive, paranoid, and conspiratorial hold over this fascist worldview. Autocratic leaders such as President Donald Trump, Vladimir Putin, and Adolf Hitler have been noted as being notoriously germophobic and fearful of contamination in private, in contrast to their public "strongman" personas (Dettmer 2020). Right-wing media outlets frequently use disease and contamination imagery to stoke fears about immigration and promote xenophobic conspiracy theories. Some researchers have found correlations between authoritarian beliefs and regional parasite- and-infectious-disease related stress (Murray et al. 2013). Right-wing paranoia around disease and illness is generally expressed in the form of anti-semitism, xenophobia, racism, and other beliefs that place the blame for infectious disease squarely on a foreign or minority "outsider" group (Bonhomme 2021).

The reason for this apparent contradiction ties back to the eugenicist beliefs that underlie fascism and other right-wing ideologies—specifically the idea that illness, disability, and social misfortune is the product of inferior genes. From this worldview, allowing COVID-19 to spread and kill people with medical vulnerabilities is akin to letting nature take its course, and purposely withholding protective public health measures to stop the spread of COVID-19 is a form of passive eugenics that accomplishes the goals of the fascist project with little required input. Surviving COVID-19 is seen as proof of physical strength and superiority (Complications? What complications?), while death and severe illness is a mark of underlying physical inferiority. From this fascist worldview, people who die or become severely ill from COVID-19 deserve their fates.

The eugenics movement and the fascist states of the early twentieth century arose in the aftermath of multiple global pandemics—all of which led to increased rates of long-term and developmental disability among survivors. People with these disabilities were marginalized within society, if not institutionalized, and blamed for the ills of a eugenicist society. Pandemics fracture societies in ways that pave the way for right-wing ideology—leading to more insular patterns of socializing, greater distrust of outgroups around disease risk specifically, and economic ripple effects that cause people to seek out an easy explanation for their misfortune. Studies surrounding the impact of the 1918 pandemic on German politics have found correlations between regional 1918 pandemic death rates and support for the Nazi Party in the 1933 German elections (Blickle 2020).

While these relationships were modest on their own, some historians suspect that these attitudes could have influenced a sufficient number of close-call local elections to allow the Nazi Party to rise to power.

Six years after the 1933 elections, the German Nazi Party issued Aktion T-4 (Rotzoll et al. 2006), a euthanasia program targeting people with disabilities, including people in institutions and children with developmental or behavioral challenges (including insufficient obedience to their parents' will). This euthanasia program was framed as a form of compassionate mercy killing but laid the groundwork for the state-sanctioned genocide of over six million Jewish and five million non-Jewish people who were seen as subhuman threats to the Nazi state.

It should come as no surprise that modern right-wing and neo-fascist ideology is incompatible with any reasonable or humane solution to the massive amount of disability caused by the COVID-19 pandemic. The rise of extreme right-wing ideology in the US and other parts of the world in the aftermath of COVID-19 has contributed to the removal of public health measures and the social safety net, increased support for white supremacist and other extremist movements, and stripped away laws that previously ensured bodily autonomy and the right to privacy for women, racial minorities, and LGBTQ+ groups. Once the impact of COVID-19 as a mass-disabling event becomes clear, this could open another avenue for recruitment into right-wing ideology, as resentment grows (and is cultivated) against people who are no longer able to work or require long-term medical services or financial assistance due to Long COVID. This represents a compounding risk to personal autonomy, democratic institutions, and societal stability itself.

4.3   HIV/AIDS and the Birth of Patient Activists

HIV/AIDS is an ongoing global pandemic that has infected an estimated 80 million people since 1980. HIV is a retrovirus that infects and destroys the immune system through the infection of the CD4 T Lymphocytes, leading to extreme susceptibility to infection and death through opportunistic cancers and infections (NIH 2021). If left untreated, HIV/AIDS is a terminal illness. However, since its initial spread in the 1980s, HIV has gone from a universally fatal condition to an illness that can be managed and even brought down to undetectable levels using antiretroviral medication.

Today, people living with HIV are able to live a relatively healthy and normal life—so long as they can maintain access to essential antiretroviral medication. The story of HIV/AIDS contains some of modern medicine and public health's greatest successes and greatest failures.

4.3.1 HIV/AIDS Patient Activism in the US

Action on HIV/AIDS in the US and other Western countries was driven primarily by a broad, diverse, and organized coalition of activists—many of whom were HIV patients themselves. In the 1980s, HIV/AIDS disproportionately spread among groups of people who were already marginalized and stigmatized by society—gay men, injection drug users, and some immigrant communities. The concentration of HIV in these "undesirable" groups contributed to the US government's lack of action and slow research on finding treatments for HIV—an instance of passive genocide that led to mass death within the LGBTQ+ community. Inaction on HIV/AIDS research and policy in the 1980s also enabled community spread of the virus outside of the initially affected communities, since people who were not members of the communities that HIV/AIDS was "supposed" to affect underestimated their personal risk and were uninformed about how to prevent transmission.

The HIV/AIDS movement in the US was led by gay men and other members of the LGBTQ+ community, who already had experience organizing and mobilizing against threats to their identities and communities. Activists within this movement tended to be young, with a latency period between their infection with the HIV virus and eventual illness and death. People who were able to devote a large amount of their time and resources to become well-known activists tended to possess wealth and social capital (e.g., wealthy, white, gay men with established professional careers). Educated and professional gay men, particularly those with a medical or scientific background, initiated the rise of the HIV patient activist movement—described by Steven Epstein in his 1995 paper on the topic as "the first social movement in the United States to accomplish the mass conversion of disease "victim" into activist-experts" (Epstein 1995).

The goal of the HIV/AIDS movement was to expedite the development and distribution of treatments for HIV by targeting federal government agencies who were seen as gatekeepers or roadblocks to these potentially lifesaving treatments (Terry 2019). These protests targeted the FDA in the early 1980s, pushing the agency to enact emergency approvals for experimental HIV drugs. HIV patient activists, who were slowly dying of a novel virus with no treatment or cure, were willing to try experimental treatments with informed consent and derided the FDA's refusal to grant this request as "paternalism."

The glacial response from the FDA in approving novel treatments for HIV did not meet the urgency of the crisis in the eyes of patients who were dying of this illness. In the late 1980s, once potential treatments were approved by the FDA and moved into clinical trials, the focus shifted to the NIH. Patients encountered many of the same issues at the NIH—existing infectious disease experts with no personal stake in the HIV crisis were poor advocates and were unwilling to bend standard clinical trial protocols to respond to the urgency of the situation. HIV patients, with their lay expertise that they had established while managing HIV/AIDS in their communities in the absence of official guidance or intervention, were not given input into clinical trials.

As a result, clinical trial participants derailed studies that prioritized "pure" scientific methodologies such as randomized control trials (RCTs) by pooling experimental and placebo medications together and distributing experimental HIV treatments obtained in these trials throughout their communities (Epstein 1998). The "pure" scientific approach that was lauded by the NIH scientists running clinical trials simply did not reflect the realities of HIV and the lives of people affected by it.

In the face of these clinical trial failures, the HIV/AIDS movement shifted its focus to establishing its members as experts on the lived experience of HIV and becoming credible enough in the eyes of the scientific establishment to become partners in research. This shift in priorities represented the birth of the patient activist movement and laid the groundwork for patient collaboration with the research enterprise. Epstein's analysis of the HIV/AIDS patient activist movement identifies four primary actions that enabled people living with HIV to obtain scientific legitimacy and become partners in the development and testing of HIV treatments:

1. **Learning the language and culture of medical science**

   HIV activists, particularly those with pre-existing scientific or medical expertise, performed deep-dive analysis on the methods of specific clinical trials and learned how issues relevant to their cause were spoken about in the biomedical research community. Activist groups who were able to speak about these issues using language and concepts familiar to researchers received a warmer reception and the willingness to listen and collaborate. The social capital of HIV/AIDS leaders who came from positions of wealth and education also played a role in bolstering their claims of credibility.

2. **Establishment of activists as representatives of the larger patient group**

   HIV/AIDS activist groups made up a small percentage of the total HIV patient population, and their politics were often more radical than those of the standard HIV patient. However, patient activists were able to convince the right authorities that they were representatives of the needs and desires of the larger patient group. The goal of this was to establish patient activists as an obligatory passage point in the recruitment of clinical trial participants. If researchers did not abide by patient advocates' requests, they could jeopardize clinical trial participation and cooperation among the communities that their patient activist research partners held sway over.

3. **Coupling of scientific and moral arguments**

   HIV patient activists advocated for specific changes to clinical trial design, such as the inclusion of more diverse patient groups, using multiple dimensions of authority. For example, a moral argument could be made for intentionally recruiting diverse clinical trial populations so that people from marginalized communities being hit hard by HIV could have early access to lifesaving treatments. It could also be argued that this same policy would increase the scientific validity of the study, and potentially identify real-world issues that would not be picked up using a mostly white, wealthy, and male sample. The linking of these arguments created a shift in how clinical trials were perceived by the research community. Prior to the HIV/AIDS pandemic, the risk inherent to clinical trial participation was seen as a burden that was unfair to force upon historically marginalized populations. HIV research reframed the clinical trial participation as a potential benefit and social good in which participants knowingly assume and consent to risk.

4. **Taking sides in pre-existing scientific debates**

   The messiness of HIV clinical trials added fuel to an existing schism in the scientific community about the value of the "gold standard" RCT and other methods that tried to cultivate "pure" science. Critics of RCTs, especially for HIV treatments, argued that the strict rules around RCT participation motivated participants to lie to researchers about trying multiple treatment approaches to maintain their participation in the trial. After all, these patients relied on their trial participation for access to lifesaving medication, while having little reason to jeopardize their lives for the "data purity" of the trial.

   Patient activists added onto this existing criticism of RCTs to push for more pragmatic and real-world-based trials that some members of the research community were already asking for. Patient activists established that people with HIV and the communities that they came from would not be easily manipulated to cater to the needs of researchers, and that designing more pragmatic studies would help find methodological common ground while addressing ethical issues.

The tireless activism of the HIV/AIDS movement forced the US and other Western governments to acknowledge the seriousness of the HIV/AIDS pandemic and changed attitudes within the scientific community toward the lived patient experience as a legitimate form of expertise, and patient groups as potential research collaborators. This pressure campaign led to the market approval of antiretroviral drugs, such as azidothymidine (AZT), in the 1990s. These treatments suppressed the replication of the HIV virus and were the first step in preventing the development of AIDS in people with HIV.

However, access to these drugs was restricted by extremely high costs set by the pharmaceutical companies who developed them and held their patent rights. Wealthy patients in Western countries could access these new treatments, but they remained out of reach for poor individuals—including all HIV patients in Africa, Asia, and other developing parts of the world where the virus was spreading rapidly.

4.3.2 HIV/AIDS Activism in the Developing World

When antiretroviral drugs became available in the 1990s, the mortality rate associated with HIV declined in Western countries, as people who could afford HIV treatment were able to maintain their health and live longer. However, as HIV/AIDS came under control in the West, the virus was exploding across the developing world, with sub-Saharan Africa being most heavily affected. The 2013 documentary *Fire In the Blood* (Mohan 2013) explores the struggle for global access to antiretroviral drugs in the late 1990s and early 2000s.

Low-income countries in the developing world were unable to afford the high prices set by Western pharmaceutical companies, whose patent protections gave them a monopoly over the price and distribution of their drugs. Drug prices were set according to Western market standards, and companies refused to reduce their prices for low-income African countries. This refusal was not out of concern for profit margins in Africa, which made up less than 1% of their total revenue, but because of fears that reducing prices in one context could cause other countries, especially large emerging markets such as China and India, to request similar discounts.

The most promising avenue for low-income African countries to be able to afford HIV medications was through lower-cost generic versions produced in countries such as India or Thailand, where no patent monopoly existed for antiretroviral drugs. However, the circumvention of the monopolies held in African countries was prohibited, with the importation of low-cost generic drugs being a criminal offense. In the 1990s, the US government and even American HIV/AIDS activists provided no assistance on this international issue, despite the rising death toll and risk to political stability posed by the unmitigated HIV pandemic.

American policy makers remained ignorant of this issue and refused to discuss it—acknowledging the disparity between the high price of HIV medications and the relatively low cost of producing them was politically risky and would raise the question of why anyone, inside the US or out, was paying so much for HIV treatment. HIV/AIDS activists feared that the forced lowering of drug prices overseas could disincentivize pharmaceutical companies from investing in HIV drug development and developing more effective medications with fewer side effects. African governments were left to deal with the HIV pandemic ravaging their people on their own.

The standoff over the manufacture and distribution of generic antiretrovirals came to a head in the early 2000s, when it became apparent that global health initiatives to combat HIV, such as the UN Global AIDS program and U.S. President's Emergency Plan for AIDS Relief (PEPFAR), would fail at their missions if they were forced to pay the price for patented antiretrovirals set by pharmaceutical companies. The solution that was finally reached was a carve-out of the Trade-Related Aspects of Intellectual Property Rights (TRIPS) agreement that exempted HIV drugs developed before 1995 from previously-mandated patent protection (CRS 2001). This carve-out finally allowed low-income countries and international aid programs to access low-cost versions of older antiretroviral drugs. However, the TRIPS agreement remained in place for any drugs developed after 1995 or in the future for HIV—or any other emergent public health crisis requiring the rapid development of new pharmaceuticals.

4.3.3 What Does HIV Have to Do with COVID?

At first glance, HIV and COVID appear to be separate global pandemics with different transmission dynamics and relatively little overlap. However, these two modern viruses have much in common—especially in their political dynamics and the patient activist movements that have mobilized around them. In his presentation *From Chronic Injustice to Health Equity* (Davids 2022), HIV activist and COVID-19 Long-hauler J. D. Davids explains the substantial interest in Long COVID that has emerged within the HIV community. HIV, even if controlled, is one of the many underlying health conditions that places people at increased risk of poor outcomes from COVID-19 infection.

People with HIV have been found to be especially at risk of developing Long COVID—one study of people who had COVID-19 prior to vaccination found the participants with HIV were four times more likely to develop Long COVID (Peluso et al. 2022). Additionally, the HIV community contains a high number of people from racial and sexual/gender minority groups, as well as disabled and other marginalized people who are at elevated risk from COVID-19. Although it poses a threat to people with HIV, COVID-19 is a type of threat that their community has previously faced and fought. The HIV community is well-organized and has decades of experience advocating around highly politicized diseases. The current struggle surrounding COVID-19 and Long COVID is the latest chapter in their long fight for health equity and disability justice.

The COVID-19 long-hauler patient activist movement is a direct descendant of ME activism and organizing, which itself draws from the patient activist model established by the HIV/AIDS movement. The HIV/AIDS, ME, and Long COVID patient activist movements share the goal of being seen as legitimate holders of expertise and research collaborators by the scientific community. As Charlotte Blease and Keith Geraghty discuss in their paper exploring accusations of "militancy" among ME patient advocates, ME (and by extension, Long COVID) patient advocates have a specific relationship with the scientific establishment that is based off the HIV/AIDS movement's engagements with these authorities (Blease and Geraghty 2018).

ME patient activists, as discussed earlier, are deeply critical of practitioners and researchers who regard ME as a psychosocial illness and promote treatments based around graded exercise or cognitive-behavioral therapy. Despite their rejection of this paradigm, much of ME activism is centered around improving and promoting meaningful patient collaboration in ME research. The desire of ME and Long COVID patients to collaborate with scientific authorities—as long as they listen to patient groups and move away from harmful illness models—is based on the model of patient activism established by the HIV/AIDS movement.

To compare the timeline of HIV/AIDS to the current circumstances with COVID-19, the situation surrounding Long COVID is most analogous to the early 1980s—prior to the development of treatments and widespread recognition of the illness outside of heavily-impacted marginalized groups. In both pandemics, patient groups were the first to document and mobilize around the novel virus, while the initial vacuum of expertise placed scientific authorities on the back foot and sowed doubt in the ability of scientific experts to respond with the urgency demanded by these unprecedented health crises (Epstein 1995). Political polarization led to both of these pandemics becoming more complex than just a medical issue, with the messy social and political dynamics embedded in these illnesses needing to be considered in any effective effort to address them.

HIV/AIDS created an exceptional policy response because of the magnitude of the crisis around the world and the high (but preventable) death rate of those affected—in addition to the tireless activism of people living with the virus. It is yet to been seen whether the human suffering and economic impact caused by Long COVID will elicit a similar sort of policy response. Despite the similarities between the two pandemics, there are also important differences that may hinder an effective policy response to Long COVID; they include the following:

1. The current lack of treatment options and uncertainty around the biological causes of Long COVID are an impediment to action on this issue that did not exist for HIV/AIDS, due to the clear relationship between the HIV virus and the disease process that it caused. The development and distribution of anti-retroviral drugs was a clear goalpost of the HIV/AIDS movement that its participants could rally around and use to pressure policy makers. A similar concrete goalpost is yet to emerge for Long COVID, although actions such as clinical trials for acute COVID treatments (i.e., Paxlovid) for long-haulers and increased funding for microclot research are potential candidates.
2. Patients who were infected with HIV, particularly those who were young and previously healthy, experienced a multi-year latency period between infection and the development of severe illness, during which they could continue to work, remain active in their communities, and participate in political demonstrations. Patients with Long COVID, by contrast, experience a comparatively rapid onset of life-limiting symptoms such as extreme fatigue, exercise intolerance, and brain fog that restrict their ability to provide and care for themselves. Long COVID patients, particularly those formerly employed in medical, legal, and other professional positions, may possess the will and expertise to collectively advocate for their cause, but face roadblocks in creating elaborate, in-person, and attention-grabbing protests due to severe fatigue being a core component of their illness.
3. The COVID-19 pandemic has taken place in a radically different information ecosystem than the HIV/AIDS movement of the 1980s and 1990s. Since this era, media consumption has moved online through increasingly fragmented and algorithm-driven social media platforms. A massive amount of information on any given topic is available to internet users, and any news story must compete for attention with this fast-moving deluge of information. Social media feeds are curated by a combination of user choice and content algorithms, and misinformation is a rampant issue that social media and content-sharing platforms such as Facebook, Twitter, WhatsApp, YouTube

and TikTok struggle to moderate. As a result, the largely grassroots online advocacy movement around Long COVID has struggled to be heard outside of the algorithmically curated information silos of people who are already informed about the condition. The low amount of coverage Long COVID has received from offline media platforms, such as TV news, has not helped the situation.

The story of the HIV/AIDS pandemic is, in many ways, a cautionary tale about healthcare inequality. Despite medical advances that have transformed HIV/AIDS from a terminal illness to a manageable condition, the HIV virus continues to spread around the world along familiar lines of inequality. The affordability and accessibility of future Long COVID diagnostics and treatments are essential components of an effective response, especially given the economic hardship imposed on individuals living with the illness. Without this consideration, few people will be able to afford treatment, and the inequalities that were laid bare by COVID-19 will become further entrenched.

References

Abdelrahman Z, Li M, Wang X (2020) Comparative review of SARS-COV-2, SARS-COV, MERS-COV, and influenza a respiratory viruses. Front. Immunol. https://doi.org/10.3389/fimmu.2020.552909

Almond D (2006) Is the 1918 Influenza pandemic over? Long-term effects of in utero influenza exposure in the post-1940 US population. Journal of Political Economy. https://www.journals.uchicago.edu/doi/abs/10.1086/507154. Accessed 20 Jan 2022

BBC (2004) Mystery of the forgotten plague. http://news.bbc.co.uk/2/hi/health/3930727.stm. Accessed 20 Jan 2022

Blease C, Geraghty K (2018) Are ME/CFS patient organizations militant? J Bio Inq 15:393–401.https://doi.org/10.1007/s11673-018-9866-5

Blickle K (2020) Pandemics change cities: Municipal spending and voter extremism in Germany, 1918–1933. Federal Reserve Bank of New York Staff Reports, no. 921. https://www.newyorkfed.org/medialibrary/media/research/staff_reports/sr921.pdf. Accessed 20 Jan 2022

Bonhomme E (2021) Germany's anti-vaccination history is riddled with anti-semitism. The Atlantic. https://www.theatlantic.com/health/archive/2021/05/anti-vaccination-germany-anti-semitism/618777/. Accessed 20 Jan 2022

Brussow H, Brussow L (2021) Clinical evidence that the pandemic from 1889 to 1891 commonly called the Russian flu might have been an earlier coronavirus pandemic. Microb Biotechnol. 14:1860–1870. https://doi.org/10.1111/1751-7915.13889

Chau S, Wong O, Ramakrishnan R (2021) History for some or lesson for all? A systematic review and meta-analysis on the immediate and long-term mental health impact of the 2002–2003 Severe Acute Respiratory Syndrome (SARS) outbreak. BMC Pub Hea. https://doi.org/10.1186/s12889-021-10701-3

Crosby A (2003) America's forgotten pandemic: The influenza of 1918 (2nd ed.). Cambridge: Cambridge University Press. https://doi.org/10.1017/CBO9780511586576

CRS (2001) HIV/AIDS drugs, patents and the trips agreement: Issues and options. Congressional Research Service. https://www.everycrsreport.com/files/20010727_RL31066_fcd08bd6166c5 e169956578611d93e73c536f423.pdf. Accessed 20 Jan 2022

Dale R, Church A, Surtees R et al (2004) Encephalitis lethargica syndrome: 20 new cases and evidence of basal ganglia autoimmunity. Brain 127:21–33. https://doi.org/10.1093/brain/awh008

Davids JD (2022) From chronic injustice to health equity (Video Communication). Massachusetts ME/CFS and Fibromyalgia. https://www.youtube.com/watch?v=MFRwkgaustY. Accessed 20 Sep 2022

Dettmer J (2020) From Putin to Bismarck, an autocrat's fear of germs. VOA News. https://www.voa news.com/a/covid-19-pandemic_putin-bismarck-autocrats-fear-germs/6191402.html. Accessed 20 Jan 2022

Eco U (1995) Ur-Fascism. https://www.pegc.us/archive/Articles/eco_ur-fascism.pdf

Epstein, S (1995) The construction of lay expertise: AIDS activism and the forging of credibility in the reform of clinical trials. Scie, Tec & Hum Val. https://www.jstor.org/stable/689868. Accessed 20 Jan 2022

Epstein S (1998) Impure science: aids, activism, and the politics of knowledge. University of California Press

JAMA (1919) Epidemic or lethargic encephalitis (NONA)72:794–795. https://doi.org/10.1001/jama. 1919.26110110001008

Kousoulis A, Tsoucalas G (2017) Infection, contagion and causality in colonial Britain: The 1889–90 influenza pandemic and the British medical journal. Infez Med. 25:285–291. https://pubmed. ncbi.nlm.nih.gov/28956550/

Lam MHB, Wing YK, Yu, MWM (2009) Mental morbidities and chronic fatigue in severe acute respiratory syndrome survivors. Arch Intern Med. 169:2142–2147. https://doi.org/10.1001/archin ternmed.2009.384

Li W, Moore M, Vasilieva N et al (2003) Angiotensin-converting enzyme 2 is a functional receptor for the SARS coronavirus. Nature 426:450–454. https://doi.org/10.1038/nature02145

Mohan GD (2013) Fire in the blood [Film]

Murray D, Schaller M, Suedfeld P (2013) Pathogens and Politics: Further Evidence That Parasite Prevalence Predicts Authoritarianism. PLOS One. https://doi.org/10.1371/journal.pone.0062275.

NIH (2021) The HIV life cycle. National Institutes of Health. https://hivinfo.nih.gov/understanding-hiv/fact-sheets/hiv-life-cycle. Accessed 20 Jan 2022

Patcai J (2022) Is long COVID similar to long SARS? Oxf Open Imm 3:1–5. https://doi.org/10.1093/ oxfimm/iqac002

Peluso M, Spinelli M, Deveau TM et al (2022) Post-acute sequelae and adaptive immune responses in people living with HIV recovering from SARS-COV-2 infection. AIDS. https://doi.org/10. 1097/QAD.0000000000003338

Rivard L (2014) America's hidden history: The eugenics movement. SciTable by Nature Education. https://www.nature.com/scitable/forums/genetics-generation/america-s-hidden-history-the-eugenics-movement-123919444/. Accessed 20 Jan 2022

Rotzoll M, Richter P, Fuchs P, et al (2006) The first national socialist extermination crime: The T4 program and its victims. International J Men Hea, 35(3), 17–29. http://www.jstor.org/stable/413 45169

Sacks O (1999) Awakenings. Vintage Books. New York City

Short K, Kedzierska K, Van de Sandt C (2018) Back to the future: Lessons learned from the 1918 influenza pandemic. Front. Cell. Infect. Microbiol. 8:343. https://doi.org/10.3389/fcimb.2018. 00343

Solly M (2020) What happened when Woodrow Wilson came down with the 1918 flu? Smithsonian Magazine. https://www.smithsonianmag.com/smart-news/what-happened-when-woodrow-wilson-came-down-1918-flu-180975972/. Accessed 20 Jan 2022

Terry M (2019) How HIV/AIDS activism led to broader patient activism in clinical trials. Biospace. https://www.biospace.com/article/how-hiv-aids-activism-led-to-broader-patient-activism-in-clinical-trials/. Accessed 20 Jan 2022

Vijgen L, Keyaerts E, Moes E (2005) Complete genomic sequence of human coronavirus oc43: molecular clock analysis suggests a relatively recent zoonotic coronavirus transmission event. J Virol. 2005 Feb; 79(3): 1595–1604. https://doi.org/10.1128/JVI.79.3.1595-1604.2005

Wilder-Smith A, Chiew C, Lee V (2020) Can we contain the COVID-19 outbreak with the same measures as for SARS? The Lancet Infectious Diseases 20:102–107. https://doi.org/10.1016/S1473-3099(20)30129-8

Zhang P, Li J, Liu H et al (2020) Long-term bone and lung consequences associated with hospital-acquired severe acute respiratory syndrome: a 15-year follow-up from a prospective cohort study. Bone Res 8:1–6. https://doi.org/10.1038/s41413-020-0084-5

.

The Threatcasting Project and Themes

5

The COVID-19 pandemic is a complex, unfolding disaster and the societal impact that its aftereffects may continue to have in the coming decades adds another layer of complexity. Between the number of people affected and the level of disability that post-COVID illness can cause, it can be staggering, if not overwhelming, to try and conceptualize what a post-COVID future will look like—let alone how to prepare for it. Attempting to draw upon historical events paints an incomplete and fragmented picture.

Although the pandemics of the past have meaningful parallels with COVID-19, no event in modern history offers a complete parallel to the downstream effects of our current pandemic. In addition to the virus itself having a wider spread and a higher rate of severe post-infection illness than any other known respiratory virus, COVID-19 exists in the context of a digitally interconnected modern society. The long-term effects of COVID-19 will almost certainly intersect with co-occurring crises such as misinformation and disinformation networks, political polarization of medicine and public health, and the climate crisis.

The goal of the pilot project that inspired this book was to try and establish a future-focused framework that can be used to conceptualize and organize the numerous impacts that Long COVID may have in the coming decades. The framework that was used for this project is Threatcasting, a scenario-planning methodology that uses interdisciplinary collaboration to model potential threats and futures in an uncertain and complex environment (Johnson et al. 2021). Threatcasting uses a workshop-based approach to identify specific, person-centered threats taking place ten years in the future from an initial event. From these threat scenarios, the group uses a process called Backcasting to discuss ways to identify, monitor, prevent, mitigate, and recover from the threat as we move forward

© The Author(s), under exclusive license to Springer Nature Switzerland AG 2024
M. Smallwood, *The Future of Long COVID*, Synthesis Lectures on Threatcasting,
https://doi.org/10.1007/978-3-031-40474-0_5

from the current moment. The goal of the workshop is to identify how to move toward a desirable future, and away from an undesirable one.

This pilot project was one of the first applications of the Threatcasting methodology to a healthcare topic. Previously, it has been used for geopolitical and national security-focused subjects, as well as for conceptualizing the unintended consequences of new and emerging technologies. However, given the level of complexity and uncertainty that exists around Long COVID, this subject proved to be a good fit for scenario planning and anticipatory foresight. Central to the Threatcasting pilot project was the input of COVID-19 long-haulers into the design of the workshop, and as participants in the workshop itself. As a participatory workshop, Threatcasting can be used as a means of patient engagement and inclusion in the discussion of complex healthcare issues. Although Long COVID stands out as a particularly complex healthcare topic with powerful future implications, a robust future-based and patient-inclusive approach could be beneficial in improving policy responses to other healthcare issues.

The Threatcasting pilot project included 25 participants, who were split between four groups—each with a similar mix of people of different backgrounds and expertise. The societal-level issues posed by Long COVID, as discussed in the threat scenarios developed and analyzed by the groups, fell into five broad categories: (1) the healthcare and mental healthcare systems, (2) disability, economics, and the workforce, (3) longitudinal impacts on children, (4) politics and politicization, and (5) the information ecosystem.

5.1   Healthcare

As a primarily medical issue, many of the long-term concerns raised about Long COVID involve aspects of the healthcare field. Most of the burden of Long COVID is expected to occur in outpatient settings, as well as increase healthcare costs and the demand for a range of medical specialties.

One overarching concern expressed by workshop participants is that the resources and attention being put toward Long COVID research are temporary and that once COVID-19 is brought under control or normalized as an endemic virus, Long COVID will fade from the public eye while millions of people continue to struggle with long-term disability. Maintaining attention and resources on the evolving needs of long-haulers, investing in longitudinal research, and continuing the beneficial healthcare accommodations made during the pandemic permanent can help sustain long-term focus on improving the quality of care for long-haulers.

5.1.1 Long COVID Education for Healthcare Providers

A patient-led survey of over 1,200 long-haulers found that during interactions with their physicians, only 18% of patients reported that their healthcare provider had a good understanding of Long COVID—while 57% reported a "poor" or "very poor" understanding. The results of this survey reflect an unfortunate reality that people with intractable forms of chronic illness have faced for years—many healthcare providers are less informed about complex chronic illnesses such as ME/CFS than their patients. The lack of provider education about these illnesses forces patients suffering from debilitating long-term symptoms to advocate for themselves and educate their providers on their conditions. Sometimes, this self-advocacy is to no avail—chronically ill patients frequently report that doctors dismiss their health concerns or attribute them to stigmatized conditions such as hypochondria, psychosomatic or psychiatric illness, and drug-seeking behavior (Guise et al. 2010). This form of dismissal is referred to as "medical gaslighting" and is especially reported among women and ethnic minority patients. Combatting these attitudes and bias within medicine is one of the most daunting, yet crucial elements of achieving progress on Long COVID and related complex chronic illnesses.

Despite the highly publicized and disruptive nature of the COVID-19 pandemic, the reported prevalence of negative provider interactions among long-haulers raises concerns that as the pandemic fades from the public eye, Long COVID will become another form of misunderstood and underdiagnosed chronic illness, despite affecting millions of people. The COVID-19 Long Haulers Act was created, in part, to address concerns over provider education by allocating $30 million to the CDC to educate healthcare providers about Long COVID.

However, this bill has not progressed past its introduction in the House of Representatives, leaving its long-term prospects uncertain. Long-haulers, alongside other chronic illness communities, have called for more education and research about multiple forms of common-but-neglected chronic illness. This call is because, instead of acting like discrete diagnostic categories, chronic illnesses such as ME/CFS, fibromyalgia, POTS, mast cell activation syndrome (MCAS), small fiber neuropathy (SFN) and others have extremely high rates of comorbidity and symptom overlap (Aaron et al. 2001).

A related area of concern brought up in the scenario-planning exercise was uncertainty over the official diagnostic criteria and standards of care for Long COVID, which had not yet been finalized at the time of the workshop. The release of this medical guidance was seen as the first step toward further policy action on Long COVID. In the year since the workshop took place, the diagnostic criteria surrounding Long COVID have been clarified and further guidance has been released, allowing for the development of medical educational materials on Long COVID. However, the dissemination of educational materials on Long COVID and complex illness to health care providers remains an ongoing issue.

5.1.2   General Awareness of Post-COVID Complications

If healthcare providers have limited knowledge of Long COVID, it is reasonable to assume that much of the American public also knows little about this new condition—or does not know that it exists at all. In summer 2022, over 90 million Americans had tested positive for COVID-19, and a substantial number of undiagnosed cases exist on top of this—with seroprevalence rates indicating that over half of Americans have had the virus at least once. Approximately one-third of the patients in post-COVID studies experience lingering symptoms—a subset of which involves long-term disability. Physiological studies of post-COVID patients have reported silent organ, endocrine, and neurological changes that were only discovered because of screening tests that were looking for these issues (Dennis et al. 2021; Mundell and Preidt 2021). If these patients had not participated in these studies, they may not have been aware of the issue or had access to the screening tools needed to diagnose it.

As the novelty and initial panic of the COVID-19 pandemic fade, and vaccination rates in wealthy countries rise, the virus is occupying a smaller part of everyday life for most Americans. While COVID-19 and Long COVID have had an impact on many American families, many more people have not experienced these threats directly. The dominant narratives surrounding COVID-19 do not acknowledge Long COVID and other medically-complex outcomes of "mild" COVID-19 cases (which do not require hospitalization). Because there is a substantial risk of medical complications from COVID-19 infection, but comparatively less public awareness that these risks exist, concern has been raised that COVID-19 could add substantial, but undiagnosed and unrecognized, medical burden across the population.

The CDC is the government agency with the most responsibility to disseminate information and raise awareness about Long COVID to the public. The COVID-19 Long Haulers Act, once passed, is intended to allocate $30 million to the CDC for Long COVID public outreach. Guidance to promote screening for common post-COVID physiological issues, such as cardiac or autonomic abnormalities, in primary care settings could increase awareness of post-COVID complications among the public, as well as provide early detection of these issues before they become serious and costly medical problems.

Some large hospital and university systems have begun to study and address the complex medical needs of post-COVID patients through post-COVID clinics. These clinics are set up to assess the symptoms of patients with Long COVID and refer them out to specialists within the same healthcare network (Young and McMahon 2020; Carbajal 2021). Currently, the demand for these clinics exceeds supply, and many clinics are dealing with long waitlists and a backlog of cases. Greater funding to expand the services and reach of post-COVID clinics would help these facilities to work through their backlog, accept new patients, and potentially play a public outreach role to raise awareness of Long COVID among the general public.

Public outreach efforts to increase awareness of Long COVID must be mindful that many ethnic minority populations that experienced disproportionately high rates of COVID exposure and infection are also underserved by healthcare and public health programs. Targeted and culturally competent public outreach to Black, Latino, and Native American communities through partnerships and funding to community-based health centers is needed to meet the needs of post-COVID patients in these populations. These partnerships should offer non-English language messaging and outreach about Long COVID, especially for communities with large immigrant populations.

The lack of public awareness around Long COVID, despite it being a condition that risks affecting millions of Americans, is a symptom of a larger culture of silence around disability. Medical conditions are common among Americans, but unless these conditions significantly impact a person's ability to work or perform everyday activities, they are generally not thought of as disabilities. The cognitive separation between disabled people and the rest of the population had fatal consequences during the COVID-19 pandemic.

The virus was initially framed as only being a threat to elderly and disabled people—a segment of the population that many people assumed was a negligible, housebound minority that could be sequestered away until the pandemic passed. In reality, the CDC estimated in August 2020 that 45.4% of American adults had at least one underlying medical condition, putting them at high risk of severe COVID-19 (Adams et al. 2020). The vulnerability of the American public to COVID-19 was exacerbated not only by the high rate of comorbid conditions but also by a severe underestimation of risk. Having more open and honest conversations about disabilities, including Long COVID, can help raise awareness of how common these issues are, and how policies surrounding them affect many Americans in ways that they might not be aware of.

5.1.3 Expanding Remote and Flexible Healthcare Options

The pandemic accelerated the adoption of virtual forms of work and communication. While technologies such as remote work, virtual conferencing, and telehealth had been rolled out for some niche uses before the pandemic, the forced, rapid retreat from in-person spaces was an incentive for workplaces in the US and across the world to quickly incorporate remote work technology into their routine functions. The healthcare field especially saw widespread adoption of telehealth during the pandemic, due to the high infection risk that in-person visits posed to medically vulnerable patients.

Telehealth has allowed the healthcare field to begin addressing long-running access issues, such as rural provider shortages and the difficulty of travel for homebound and chronically ill patients. Telehealth expansion was enabled by temporary pandemic-era policies that loosened restrictions and increased Medicare and Medicaid coverage of remote doctors' visits (Koma et al. 2021). Policy actions to make these temporary expansions to telehealth coverage permanent could have a substantial impact on increasing healthcare access to underserved communities that have been disproportionately impacted by the pandemic. Resolving regulatory issues with telehealth and improving broadband and wireless infrastructure in rural and impoverished communities are also necessary steps to enabling long-term telehealth expansion.

The pandemic has also renewed calls for the expansion of home-based and palliative care for patients newly disabled by Long COVID, patients with disabling conditions such as diabetes and kidney failure, and elderly people who wish to remain in their homes. Palliative care is a type of home-based care that is focused on symptom management instead of rehabilitation from an illness or injury. People with non-terminal chronic illness argue that access to this form of care could greatly improve their quality of life while reducing the stress placed on family members in caretaker roles.

However, people with long-term chronic illnesses often experience difficulty obtaining insurance coverage for home-based and palliative forms of care. Many forms of insurance, including Medicare, only cover palliative services in the form of hospice care for patients that are expected to be in their last six months of life (Ollove 2021). The widespread disability caused by the COVID-19 pandemic bolsters the argument that home-based and palliative healthcare needs to be expanded and covered by insurance beyond just patients in their last months of life. A higher number of non-elderly people who will be requiring this level of long-term care is an unfortunate reality of a world with widespread Long COVID. However, allowing people to receive these services in their homes will reduce the load on other parts of the healthcare system, and allow people to receive care with greater safety and dignity.

5.1.4 Addressing the Provider Shortage

The predicted rise in demand for healthcare services as a result of Long COVID and other post-COVID medical complications is occurring simultaneously with staffing shortages at hospitals and other healthcare institutions. The heavy strain placed on hospital systems by the COVID-19 pandemic has resulted in the death, disabling (including through Long COVID), burnout, and resignation of nurses, doctors, and other healthcare professionals, leading to widespread concern about the sustainability of the healthcare system.

The anticipated healthcare needs of the Long COVID population differ somewhat from the areas of healthcare most impacted by acute COVID-19. While the COVID-19 pandemic hit hospital systems with a large volume of patients requiring intensive care, the healthcare needs of long-haulers are expected to primarily require outpatient care. Within an outpatient setting, the complex and multi-systemic symptoms of Long COVID mean that patients are often referred to multiple specialists, with primary care and general practitioners being unable to provide much guidance due to their unfamiliarity with the condition.

Workforce development practices that bring additional staff into needed specialties and provide current practitioners with continuing education on Long COVID can help expand the pool of providers who can provide adequate care for Long COVID patients. Providing additional funding for post-COVID clinics can also increase the efficiency of care for patients requiring the care of multiple specialists and reduce encounters with medical practitioners who are uninformed about Long COVID.

5.1.5 Dealing with Insurance Denials

The Affordable Care Act (ACA) prohibits health insurance discrimination against people with pre-existing conditions. However, there is no law prohibiting providers of life, disability, or long-term care insurance from underwriting pre-existing conditions to charge higher premiums or deny coverage. Insurance risk assessors tasked with monitoring the consequences of the COVID-19 pandemic have been among the most diligent followers of new developments with Long COVID. Some insurers not only classify Long COVID as a pre-existing condition, but consider any documented COVID-19 infection to be a risk factor for future medical complications (Price and Vardavas 2020).

Life insurance policy denials based on a positive COVID-19 test, even for people with mild or asymptomatic cases, have been reported since 2020 (Wheeler 2020). Extremely high rates of disability insurance denial for Long COVID claims have also been reported, with the appeals process for these denials being deliberately time-intensive (Vogel 2021). Currently, there is little to no legal protection—barring legislative action—against this type of underwriting for Americans who have tested positive for COVID-19. Diligent surveillance and additional documentation of such instances of discrimination may help build the case for legislative action on this issue.

5.1.6 Mental Healthcare

Dealing with the neurological and psychiatric impacts of Long COVID was an issue that multiple groups in the Threatcasting group took interest in and chose as a scenario prompt. This interest was likely due to the triple impact that the aftereffects of COVID-19 pose to the behavioral health system:

1. The subtype of Long COVID known as "neurocovid," in which sufferers experience cognitive dysfunction, brain fog, depression, anxiety, and even dementia-like symptoms, as well as other structural changes and pathologies observed in the brains of post-COVID patients (Douaud et al. 2021);
2. The increased risk of depression, suicidality, and other mental health issues for people experiencing Long COVID symptoms that limit their everyday functioning; and

3. The increased rates of depression and anxiety observed among the general population
   during the pandemic.

Many of the concerns raised about the impact of Long COVID on the behavioral health
system focus on the chronic underfunding and neglect of mental health—including
provider shortages, substandard care for non-acute mental health concerns, and a lack
of reliable insurance coverage (Altiraifi and Rapfogel 2020). Addressing these concerns
in the context of Long COVID is a component of the long-running push to improve access
to appropriate mental healthcare for millions of Americans.

An area of concern that is specific to Long COVID and related chronic illnesses is the
need to assess the appropriate mental healthcare required for these populations. People
experiencing long-term chronic illness are at high risk for mental distress, low self-
reported quality of life, and suicidal ideation for a combination of reasons—some being
related to the life-limiting qualities of their illness, and others being due to a lack of social
support (Chu et al. 2021). Appropriate behavioral health interventions can help chronic
illness patients deal with some components of their illness, such as depression and sleep
disturbances. However, there is a long history of tension and distrust between chronic
illness patients and the behavioral health system due to ignorance and misunderstandings
about these complex chronic health conditions (Guise et al. 2010).

When practitioners do not have a good understanding of such health conditions,
frequent reporting of symptoms with no apparent biological cause is often attributed
to stigmatized psychiatric or psychosomatic causes—essentially dismissing a patient's
concerns as "being all in their head." To adequately address the mental health needs
of post-COVID patients, behavioral health practitioners need to be educated about the
complex nature of Long COVID and understand how the coexisting psychiatric and
bodily symptoms of post-COVID patients are intertwined, yet distinct. Better education
about chronic illness among behavioral health practitioners is an important first step in
establishing trust and providing appropriate mental health treatment for long-haulers.

5.2   Disability, Employment and Economics

In addition to apprehension over the ability of the healthcare system to provide sufficient
healthcare for post-COVID patients, an area of concern that was discussed in nearly every
threat scenario was the ability of Long COVID patients to remain autonomous, housed,
employed (if possible), or otherwise economically-supported. The points raised about
the economic implications of Long COVID fell into two main, interrelated categories—
the need to insulate long-haulers from economic ruin and a loss of autonomy, and the
compounded impacts of Long COVID on employers and the labor force if the former
need was not met.

The economic risks posed to individuals by Long COVID are similar to those faced by people with other types of long-term disability and are exacerbated by the weakening of the social safety net. However, the disruptions to the workforce caused by the pandemic and other patterns of technological and social change may cause—or force—employers to reimagine standard workplace practices. The permanent adoption of remote work, expansion of wages and health benefits, and normalization of flexibility and accommodation within the workplace are labor trends that can enable some long-haulers to remain employed and autonomous.

5.2.1   Reducing the Burden on Families

When policy decisions fail to allow people with disabilities to live independently, the responsibility of care falls on family members. These situations increase the risk of negative outcomes for disabled individuals and their family members alike—including loss of individual autonomy, strained family relationships, increased risk of domestic violence and other forms of abuse, and greater economic hardship. The burden of forced caretaking for families who cannot afford other support options also reduces the number of available workers in the labor market, since individuals with caregiving responsibilities to an ill relative often do not have the time or energy to work a standard job.

The burden of caretaking roles during the pandemic has disproportionately fallen on women, who have been unable to return to the labor force at the same rate as their male counterparts (Madgavkar et al. 2020). Policy actions aimed at providing economic support for people with Long COVID should work to prioritize individual well-being and reduce the caretaking responsibilities borne by family members. Expansion of home and community-based services (HBCS) and the funding of these services through Medicare and Medicaid, as discussed in Chap. 2, is an important part of reducing the caretaking responsibilities being taken up by unprepared family members.

5.2.2   Reforming Supplemental Security Income (SSI)

SSI is the main program through which the US government provides economic support to individuals with disabilities that render them unable to work. Approximately eight million Americans rely on SSI for survival, and concerns have long been raised by disability rights advocates about the program's poverty-level payouts and the strict lifestyle restrictions that the program imposes on individuals (CBPP 2018). As of 2022, SSI pays $841 per month to individuals, and $1,261 to couples (SSA 2022)—a rate that is insufficient to account for inflation and the cost of living in many parts of the country (Altiraifi 2020).

The reduced SSI payout to couples imposes harsh penalties on disabled people for marrying—risking either a drastic cut in the couple's combined monthly payment or losing benefits altogether and becoming financially dependent on their spouse.

Perhaps the most derided aspect of SSI by disability rights advocates is the $2,000 asset limit—a rule that forces disabled people to live in poverty and prohibits them from saving extra money for emergencies. Even short-term increases to a checking or savings account, such as a well-intentioned gift from a friend or relative, have led to cases of disabled people losing their SSI or Medicaid eligibility (Turkewitz and Linderman 2012). The Achieving a Better Life Experience Act (ABLE) account program, launched in 2016, has taken steps to remedy the asset account issue by allowing people on SSI to save up to $100,000 for medical expenses through the program. However, this program is only available to people whose documented disability began before age 26 (ABLE National Resource Center 2021).

The SSI Restoration Act of 2021, which would take steps to increase SSI payouts to 100% of the federal poverty line; raise the asset limit to $10,000 for individuals and $20,000 for couples; and update or eliminate SSI rules that penalize individuals for marrying, earning supplemental income, or receiving family support; has been introduced in the Senate (US Congress 2021). However, little action has been taken on the bill since its introduction, and it faces an uphill battle in being able to pass the Senate vote.

5.2.3 Accommodating Long-Haulers in the Workforce

The problems associated with SSI strengthen the argument for policymakers and private employers alike to ensure that people experiencing long-term medical complications from COVID-19 can remain in the workforce. For some long-haulers, a technology enabling them to keep their jobs while managing their health already exists—remote work. Remote work was a nearly ubiquitous tool used by some segments of the workforce during the pandemic with mixed reception. While some workers employed in information-based office jobs missed the social contact afforded by the office, other workers, including many with disabilities, greatly appreciated the increased flexibility that working from home provided. As vaccination has allowed more workers to safely return to in-person work, a fight has emerged between employees who want—or need—to keep working remotely, and employers who are mandating a return to in-person work.

Among the employees advocating for permanent remote work are people who developed Long COVID during the pandemic. They argue that they were only able to maintain both their health and their jobs due to the flexibility that remote work enables. These employed long-haulers worry that if they are forced to return to in-person work and the physical stressors associated with it—such as commuting, long working hours, and schedule inflexibility—they will no longer be able to maintain this balance and may be forced to quit their jobs (Maldonado 2021). One proposed solution for this dilemma is to establish remote work as a reasonable accommodation for disabled workers under the Americans with Disabilities Act (ADA).

This would require employers to accommodate the remote work needs of long-haulers who request this accommodation. However, using the ADA to allow some people to continue working remotely only addresses the issue on an individual, rather than a systemic level. Requesting accommodations requires an employee to advocate for themselves and provide proof of disability to their employer—an act that can jeopardize their employment or chances for career advancement, despite laws against this sort of discrimination. A broader solution would be to normalize remote work as a viable work option—a policy that many prominent companies in the technology sector, such as Slack and Adobe, are choosing to adopt (Stoller 2021). Cost–benefit analysis and employee advocacy could provide additional motivation for companies to maintain remote work options, since the flexibility offered by remote work can be beneficial for workers with a variety of needs, and may help employers maintain their existing workforce. Workplace consultants could help companies resolve issues with the logistics of transitioning to remote or hybrid work.

Much of the existing discussion over accommodating the needs of long-haulers in the workplace is centered around workers whose jobs can be performed remotely, such as those with office, clerical, or information-based jobs. However, many jobs, such as healthcare, construction, agricultural, food service, and retail work, require in-person attendance. Workers in these jobs do not have the option of remote work and are more likely to have been exposed to COVID-19 during the pandemic, and in some cases, are not provided with healthcare and other benefits.

Compared to office-based workers, there is far less conversation and potentially fewer solutions to accommodating long-term disabilities from COVID-19 infection in this part of the workforce. Efforts to raise wages, offer benefits, and improve working conditions may help some workers with COVID-19 related medical complications, but the physical component of these jobs may force some workers with Long COVID to quit—possibly without other viable employment options. Some long-haulers may be able to use job retraining programs to find more accommodating forms of employment, but fatigue or cognitive issues may prove to be barriers for others.

5.2.4   Working Toward Systemic Solutions

The COVID-19 pandemic exposed long-running issues and inequality in the US that have been worsened by the weakening of social safety net programs. Many public programs that are designed to provide services to people in need exist within the federal and state governments. However, they are often underfunded, understaffed, and—despite high demand for their services—underutilized by populations who could benefit from them. In her article "The Time Tax," Anne Lowrey (2021) explores how public assistance programs are designed to have complicated and time-intensive application processes that discourage people who might otherwise qualify for assistance from applying.

The end goal of this intentional design process is to reduce the number of applicants and the cost of the program. However, this type of labyrinthine application process is only seen in public programs that are targeted toward a specific, disadvantaged subset of the population, such as Medicaid, TANF, SNAP, SSI, and unemployment. Where this complex application process is not seen is in public programs that apply to a broad population, such as Medicare and Social Security. These sorts of public programs also tend to have high public approval ratings, and efforts to restrict or complicate them are deeply unpopular.

In the context of addressing Long COVID and other aspects of recovering from the COVID-19 pandemic, it is important to keep in mind that while programs targeting the needs of specific disadvantaged groups are important, they are also politically vulnerable and may be set up for failure if the services are unable to help the people in need of them. Broad improvements to the social safety net may be politically popular and resilient, and may also help the larger group of people who experience complications from COVID-19, but who don't qualify for—or aren't aware of—specialized assistance programs.

5.3   Longitudinal Impact on Children

The workshops for this project were conducted in August 2021—during the Delta surge and the heated societal discussion over a return to in-person schooling. In the first year of the pandemic, prior to the emergence of the highly infectious Delta variant, COVID-19 posed the highest level of risk to older adults, with children and teenagers being comparatively unlikely to be hospitalized or experience severe outcomes. This early demographic pattern contributed to the belief that children are not vulnerable to COVID-19, and that the primary argument for closing in-person schools was to prevent children from spreading the virus to older and more vulnerable members of their families and communities.

Once vaccines became available to the adult population in 2021, there was intense political pressure to return to in-person schooling—despite the fact that children could not yet be vaccinated against COVID-19. The return to in-person schooling during the peak of the Delta variant, combined with low community vaccination rates and bans on mask mandates in many Republican-ruled states, has raised concerns about the long-term developmental impacts of COVID-19 infection among unvaccinated children.

Many groups in the workshop were interested in this issue, and developed scenarios centered around people who developed long-term complications from COVID-19 as children or teenagers and suffered from poor academic performance and an inability to transition into higher education or the workforce as a result. Since the winter of 2021–2022—when the rapid spread of the Omicron variant resulted in mass infection of the younger age groups that had been spared from earlier waves of the pandemic—many of the issues raised around Long COVID and children have become far less hypothetical.

5.3.1 Direct Impacts of COVID-19

Although the common belief that children and teenagers are less likely than older adults to experience severe outcomes from COVID-19 is true in a general sense, it leaves many of the most vulnerable children in our society out of the conversation. A disproportionate number of Black and Hispanic children are represented in data monitoring deaths, severe illness, and Multi-System Inflammatory Syndrome (MIS). Most children who have died from COVID-19 had at least one pre-existing diagnosis, the most common ones being obesity, asthma, and developmental disorders (McCormick et al. 2021).

The disproportionate risk of severe COVID-19 faced by people with disabilities, compared to the relatively low risk to the non-disabled population, has been used throughout the pandemic to argue against public health measures that impose rules and restrictions on the behavior of healthy individuals at low risk for severe illness. This argument not only presents the deaths of people with disabilities and underlying health conditions as acceptable casualties in the pursuit of personal freedom, but also assumes that comorbidities that increase the risk of severe COVID-19 are rare occurrences among the American population.

The reality is that these underlying health conditions are common in the US, including among the pediatric population. The two main risk factors for severe pediatric COVID-19 outcomes—obesity and asthma—affect 19.3% (CDC 2021c) and 7% (CDC 2021b) of children in the US respectively, with Black, Hispanic, Native American, and children from low-income families being over-represented in these numbers (CDC 2021d). The risk posed by COVID-19 infection to children with disabilities has been the subject of multiple lawsuits against Republican governors who have prohibited school mask mandates.

These lawsuits argue that prohibiting universal masking in schools, an effective but politically volatile COVID-19 prevention measure, violates the ADA by denying children at high risk of severe COVID-19 a safe environment in which to obtain an equal education to their peers (Disability Rights Texas 2021b). In November 2021, the federal court hearing the case brought against a Texas law banning mask mandates in schools ruled in favor of the plaintiffs, stating that policies that prohibit schools from enforcing mask mandates to protect high-risk children from COVID-19 are in violation of the ADA (Disability Rights Texas 2021a).

Beyond the risks that COVID-19 infection poses to children with underlying health conditions, numerous concerns have been raised about the long-term consequences of COVID infection in children and teenagers. Preliminary data from the UK found that between 10–15% of surveyed children experienced at least one lingering symptom five weeks after infection, compared to 25% of adults in the same study (Ayoubkhani et al. 2021). A study of children infected with COVID in Israel showed similar figures—approximately 10% experienced lingering symptoms (Israel Ministry of Health 2021). However, diagnosing Long COVID in pediatric patients may be more difficult than in adults. Many common symptoms of Long COVID, such as fatigue and brain fog, rely on patient self-reporting and do not possess reliable biomarkers.

Children may not have the language or body awareness to explain their symptoms in detail the way an adult patient might. One example of this, described by *Long COVID Families* founder Megan Carmilani, is that adults with Long COVID can use their pre-COVID state of health as a baseline to put the severity of their symptoms into perspective. Children who develop Long COVID at a young age, on the other hand, may not be able to conceptualize such a baseline due to having less life experience (Carmilani 2022). Children also have diminished autonomy compared to adults and are reliant on their caretakers for access to medical care. This represents an additional barrier to care for children whose parents cannot afford access to medical care, or who subscribe to COVID-19 misinformation and do not believe that Long COVID exists.

Even if children are less likely than adults to develop Long COVID, they still represent a significant portion of the current cohort of young people who may experience lifelong health problems, academic difficulties, and a reduced ability to thrive. The long-term developmental impacts of COVID-19 infection are unknown, but brain imaging studies that show silent organ damage, gray matter loss, and permanent changes to brain structure in post-COVID patients raise concerns about future physical and psychiatric disability (Douaud et al. 2021).

Many of the questions pertaining to the long-term impact of COVID infection on children require further research to elucidate the scope of this problem. Post-COVID studies that examine the pediatric population specifically need to be designed, instead of assuming that research conducted with adult cohorts will be applicable to children as well. Pediatricians need to be included in conversations about post-COVID standards of care, and the medical community must acknowledge that Long COVID and post-COVID complications can and do affect children, instead of being perceived as an illness observed only in adult populations.

5.3.2 Indirect Impacts of COVID-19

Children and teenagers are, in general, less vulnerable to poor outcomes from COVID-19 infections than adults. However, they are more vulnerable to the indirect effects and stressors that the pandemic has inflicted upon families, such as caregiver death, illness, unemployment, eviction, and homelessness. The NIH estimates that over 140,000 children in the US—1 in 500—have lost a caregiver to COVID-19, and that ethnic minority families make up 65% of families affected by caregiver death.

The economic disruption caused by the pandemic and subsequent recession also increased financial instability and caused many families to fall behind on rent or be unable to afford food or other expenses (CBPP 2021). Some pandemic-era policies, such as expanded unemployment benefits, eviction moratoriums, and the Expanded Child Tax

Credit were able to insulate families from poverty, eviction, and homelessness throughout 2020 and early 2021. However, the expiration and non-renewal of these policies means that many children and families who were initially protected from the worst economic impacts of the pandemic again face an uncertain future.

The indirect effects of the pandemic on children are a cause for concern due to the cumulative impact that chronic forms of childhood stress—commonly known as Adverse Childhood Experiences (ACEs)—have on long-term health outcomes. Stressors such as caregiver death, family poverty, eviction, or homelessness are considered extremely serious risk factors for the development of long-term physical and mental health problems (CDC 2021a). Protective factors such as family and community stability can help children recover from toxic stressors.

To prevent pandemic-era stressors—caregiver loss and economic stress—from manifesting into long-term health problems, policies to address these issues should focus on providing financial and emotional support to affected families, ensuring surviving families can stay together, and increasing community strength and support. One major hurdle to these policies is the lack of a centralized system to keep track of children who have been orphaned or impacted by COVID-19—much of the existing support for these children and their families is provided through disparate local organizations.

5.4 Politics and Politicization

The COVID-19 pandemic has been deeply politicized since its start in the US—in large part due to the general polarization and politicization of formerly neutral topics observed during the tenure of former President Donald Trump. The politicization of COVID-19, vaccines, and public health measures has continued due to widespread misinformation and the opposition to public health measures being adopted as a core component of political identity by a significant portion of the Republican Party.

The politicization of COVID-19, as well as the overall American political system, presents two main concerns regarding Long COVID—federal inaction, particularly on the Congressional level, and a patchwork of policies enacted by state governments—raising uncertainty over whether the proposed policies to address the needs of long-haulers have a realistic chance of becoming law. Additionally, COVID misinformation, conspiracy theories, and political radicalization among the public has continued to be a problem into 2021 and 2022, and much of this right-wing political movement exists on a decentralized, local level that is difficult to monitor or control.

5.4.1 Political Inaction and Dysfunction

From the spring of 2021 to the summer of 2022, the Senate was stuck in negotiation over a high-profile budget reconciliation bill originally meant to provide $3.5 trillion to a broad range of programs needed to help the US recover from the COVID-19 pandemic—and the long-running systemic issues that exacerbated it. The bill, which was finally signed in August of 2022 as the Inflation Reduction Act, was an ambitious social spending bill that had to passed with unanimous consent from Democratic senators—due to the tense political dynamics of the 117th Congress's evenly divided senate and the refusal of all Senate Republicans to support the bill.

The drawn-out negotiations over the contents of the bill resulted in many of the policies and funding priorities originally promised in the bill being cut or given reduced funding. The fight over the Inflation Reduction Act was seen by many as only the latest incident in a pattern of congressional dysfunction that draws into question the viability of passing any effort to expand the social safety net into law. The creation of new social safety net programs, or the expansion of existing ones, is often tied to other politically volatile legislation, and can fail for reasons unrelated to that program or the need it fills.

In the absence of federal policy in 2021 and 2022, decisions regarding local aspects of COVID-19 recovery were dictated at the state level. The political polarization over COVID-19 response by state governors and legislatures resulted in a patchwork approach to the pandemic across the country. Many blue states encouraged policies such as mask mandates, vaccination, increased unemployment assistance, and restrictions on eviction, while some red states enacted policies opposing these measures with the goal of prioritizing a return to the pre-pandemic status quo—such as prohibiting mask mandates, using pandemic relief funds for other purposes, and refusing to expand access to Medicaid and unemployment assistance. This created reasonable concern about the fates of long-haulers living in states whose governments had objected to mitigating the virus from the early stage of the pandemic.

However, since 2022, the political narrative of the pandemic has shifted towards normalizing the spread of the virus and returning to pre-pandemic patterns of behavior—a push towards 'living with the virus' that has been embraced by members of both political parties. This evolution of the narrative has pushed funding for public health mitigations out of the government's hands, and towards the private market—with high-risk individuals being advised to take individual level precautions instead of relying on institutional accommodations. In a sense, this shift in the narrative has diminished COVID's status as a point of political contention between the two dominant political parties. While still politically-charged, it has become an issue that neither political party has the will to take continued action on.

It is no understatement to say the that people who have suffered great personal loss from the pandemic—including those who have lost their health to Long COVID or who are otherwise high-risk for severe COVID complications—feel abandoned by this shift in policy. There is substantial concern among these groups that as the virus continues spreading and evolving—leaving variable forms of disability in its wake—that nothing short of another mass-casualty event will be able revive mainstream political interest in tackling the long tail of the pandemic. The future of Long COVID and the people living with it is deeply entangled with the need for continued political awareness and action on the long-term effects of the pandemic—even as this fight appears to be an increasingly uphill battle. Examples of policy actions that focus has shifted towards include widespread upgrades of ventilation and filtration in buildings, to control the spread of the virus in the absence of other mitigations, and pressuring states with unused pandemic relief funds to direct these resources towards Long COVID clinics and care. To avoid the worst long-term outcomes of the pandemic, political pressure needs to be sustained on actions to reduce the spread of the virus and build capacity within the healthcare and social safety net systems to absorb the increased rates of disability that are, unfortunately, already baked in.

5.4.2 Politicization of Public Health

Extreme political polarization over COVID-19 and anything related to it has exacerbated the spread of the virus and the extension of the pandemic in the US. Many of the public actions opposing COVID prevention measures, such as vaccinations and mask mandates, have taken place on a local level, and have involved protests, political pressure, and even death threats aimed at local officials such as school boards, city councils, and public health officials.

In response to this political pressure, elected officials in Republican-leaning states and regions disregarded pre-existing public health response plans and recommendations from federal advisory agencies such as the CDC in favor of ideologically-driven policies that have increased the spread of the virus. As of 2022, many Democratic-led states and federal advisory agencies such as the CDC have capitulated to these same political pressures and have implicitly or explicitly admitted that continued acknowledgment and mitigation of COVID-19 and its aftereffects are politically charged topics.

Political radicalization against public health measures is a difficult and intractable problem to solve, and it shows little sign of reversing course as the pandemic drags on. Steps to alleviate this issue at the state level include efforts to depoliticize public health, adhere to existing response plans in future outbreaks, and research the local economic impacts of the pandemic. However, these changes will require buy-in from state and local elected officials—something that is by no means guaranteed in the current political environment. Addressing anti-public health sentiment among the public poses additional challenges, due to the decentralized nature of the problem. In many cases, these attitudes are being fueled by online misinformation on large, unregulated social media networks such as Facebook,

Twitter, Reddit, and TikTok. This is a broad problem that policymakers are trying, and struggling, to manage.

5.5   Information Ecosystem

The pandemic drove large segments of the population online, with the internet being their primary source of information, communication, and socialization. This had both positive and negative impacts. The coalescence of COVID-19 survivors through social media led to the creation and eventual widespread recognition of Long COVID as a real medical condition with significant public health implications. However, these same online platforms were a conduit for the spread of misinformation, conspiracy theories, and political radicalization for other segments of the population. Online misinformation is being increasingly recognized as an emerging threat—but one that is difficult to directly combat due to its decentralized nature.

5.5.1   Long COVID-Specific Scams and Misinformation

People with chronic illnesses such as Long COVID and ME/CFS face significant challenges in taking part in aspects of everyday life—particularly those that require in-person attendance, travel, or physical exertion. Because of this, long-haulers may come to rely on the internet for much of their information and social interaction—even more heavily than the general population. This raises concerns over whether long-haulers—particularly those experiencing cognitive impairments from their illness—may be at higher risk for exposure to online misinformation or scams targeting people with long-term health problems.

The lack of clinically approved diagnostics and treatments for Long COVID and the vacuum of authority that this has created around the illness (as discussed in Sect. 3.1.2) means that Long COVID patients could be a major target for people looking to profit from the sale of unproven medical treatments. The risk of emerging Long COVID medical scams is compounded by the wide and variable range of symptoms that long-haulers experience, and the desperation of many patients to obtain any form of relief.

Misinformation and scams surrounding Long COVID have yet to be the subject of inquiry for researchers or federal investigators. Peer support groups and online long-hauler networks, particularly those with scientifically-literate members, currently provide a buffer against predatory scams and misinformation for people connected to these networks. However, the information and fact-checking being shared through these online networks has had limited success in being disseminated to the wider population.

People experiencing post-COVID symptoms who are not aware of Long COVID or connected to peer support networks are at particularly high risk of falling victim to health-related scams. People put in this position, who often have pre-existing risk factors such as old age, cognitive disability, or social isolation, are reluctant to report scams due to feelings of shame and embarrassment. This fact, unfortunately, makes identifying and prosecuting scammers even more difficult for law enforcement and consumer protection agencies. More pre-emptive vigilance by agencies such as the Bureau of Consumer Protection (BCP) toward Long COVID's potential to become a hotbed for medical scams could help protect long-haulers from becoming targets of predatory misinformation. Collaborations between the BCP and long-hauler communities could help investigators catch emerging scams early on and serve as a buffer that may encourage people targeted by scams to come forward.

5.5.2 Broader Action on Misinformation

Much of the concern over the information ecosystem expressed during the Threatcasting workshop dealt with the role of the internet in spreading misinformation, conspiracy theories, and extreme political ideologies. Concerns over the real-world effects of online misinformation existed prior to the pandemic, but public conversation over the issue gained new momentum during the multiple crises that came to define the year 2020.

Online misinformation is a difficult, often intractable problem to combat as it often spreads in decentralized, informal, and insulated online spaces, such as Facebook groups and message boards such as Reddit. People who believe online misinformation do not respond to fact-based counter-arguments—while the ideas that they believe may be false, their reasons for believing in it are often tied to an emotional or ideological core instead of a logical one (Moyer 2019). Misinformation is not a new issue, but the way in which the internet has allowed it to spread rapidly and with little external oversight is an unprecedented issue that experts are struggling to gain a handle on.

One way that policymakers are currently trying to reduce the spread of misinformation is through regulating the social media platforms that these ideas spread through. Some of the actions that have been proposed to disrupt misinformation networks, such as stricter content moderation and the termination of accounts that are major misinformation nodes, require the cooperation of the private companies that own platforms such as Facebook (Kang 2021). Such interventions may only be temporary solutions with unintended consequences—misinformation networks may simply move to other websites that will not restrict their content, while stricter content moderation may be used as a back door to censor other forms of online political speech (West 2017).

Efforts to identify what counts as COVID-19 or Long COVID misinformation—and who makes this call—also has the potential to backfire. The rapid spread of the Omicron variant, the dismantling of public COVID-19 testing infrastructure, and sudden changes in the CDC's metrics for communicating community risk levels (Stone 2022) has made questions about what the "real" COVID-19 data is increasingly murky. As the split widens between the "official" narrative on COVID-19 and people who believe that this narrative downplays the number of cases and risk associated with the virus, efforts to communicate risk that go against the dominant narrative may themselves be flagged as misinformation.

Online misinformation on COVID-19 is one of the most difficult and intractable issues of the pandemic to address, and the problem is becoming worse as competing narratives about the virus circulate. The spread of harmful and false information online through informal social media networks should also regarded as a serious threat by people who work in risk assessment. Efforts to create response plans for future crises need to take into account the fact that a significant minority of the public may not believe that the crisis is a real threat due to exposure to online misinformation.

5.5.3 Cybersecurity

A final issue discussed in several of the workshop scenarios deals with larger concerns over healthcare infrastructure. When the Threatcasting workshop was conducted, several high-profile ransomware attacks against hospital systems, sanitation networks, and municipal governments had recently been in the news. In 2020, an analysis by Emsisoft found that 2,354 entities in the US experienced ransomware attacks—560 of which were healthcare facilities (Davis 2021). The FBI and other federal law enforcement agencies are currently underequipped to investigate and resolve every ransomware case. In many attacks, especially those targeting medical and municipal infrastructure, the targets are forced to pay the ransom to quickly restore vital services (Nakashima et al. 2021).

The recent prominence of ransomware attacks on healthcare providers, combined with the movement toward electronic medical recordkeeping, has raised concerns about the security of medical records—especially for people with long medical histories and complex conditions that require communication between multiple providers. The question whether the strengthening of online infrastructure should be funded in the same way as more traditional forms of physical infrastructure is currently a point of debate within Congress. However, as prominent malware attacks have shown, these two types of infrastructure can be deeply intertwined.

References

Aaron L, Herrell R, Ashton S et al (2001) Comorbid clinical conditions in chronic fatigue. J Gen Intern Med. 16:24–31. https://doi.org/10.1111/j.1525-1497.2001.03419.x

ABLE National Resource Center (2021) About able accounts. National Disability Institute. https://www.ablenrc.org/what-is-able/what-are-able-acounts/. Accessed 20 Jan 2022

Adams M, Katz D, Grandpre J (2020) Population-based estimates of chronic conditions affecting risk for complications from coronavirus disease, united states. Emerging Infectious Diseases 26(8): Aug 2020. https://wwwnc.cdc.gov/eid/article/26/8/20-0679_article. Accessed 20 Jan 2022

Altiraifi A, Rapfogel N (2020) Mental health care was severely inequitable, then came the coronavirus crisis. Center for American Progress. https://www.americanprogress.org/issues/disability/reports/2020/09/10/490221/mental-health-care-severely-inequitable-came-coronavirus-crisis/. Accessed 20 Jan 2022

Altiraifi, A (2020) A deadly poverty trap: Asset limits in the time of the coronavirus. Center for American Progress. https://www.americanprogress.org/article/deadly-poverty-trap-asset-limits-time-coronavirus/. Accessed 20 Jan 2022

Ayoubkhani D, Bosworth M, King S (2021) Prevalence of ongoing symptoms following coronavirus (COVID-19) infection in the UK. United Kingdom Office for National Statistics. https://www.ons.gov.uk/peoplepopulationandcommunity/healthandsocialcare/conditionsanddiseases/datasets/alldatarelatingtoprevalenceofongoingsymptomsfollowingcoronaviruscovid19infectionintheuk. Accessed 20 Jan 2022

Carbajal E (2021) 44 hospitals, health systems that have launched post-COVID-19 clinics. Becker's Hospital Review. https://www.beckershospitalreview.com/patient-safety-outcomes/13-hospitals-health-systems-that-have-launched-post-covid-19-clinics.html. Accessed 20 Jan 2022

Carmilani M (2022) The global interdependence center—solve long COVID initiative program series: Session III: Long COVID and children (Video Communication). Global Interdependence Center. https://www.interdependence.org/resources/the-global-interdependence-center-solve-long-covid-initiative-program-series-session-iii-long-covid-and-children/#.yw_1r3bmk. Accessed 20 Sep 2022

CBPP (2018) Supplemental security income (SSI). Center on Budget and Policy Priorities. https://www.cbpp.org/research/social-security/supplemental-security-income-ssi. Accessed 20 Jan 2022

CBPP (2021) Tracking the COVID-19 Economy's Effects on Food, Housing, and Employment Hardships. Center on Budget and Policy Priorities. https://www.cbpp.org/sites/default/files/atoms/files/8-13-20pov.pdf. Accessed Sep 2022

CDC (2021a) Adverse childhood experiences (ACES). Centers for Disease Control and Prevention. https://www.cdc.gov/vitalsigns/aces/index.html. Accessed 20 Jan 2022

CDC (2021b) Asthma. Centers for Disease Control and Prevention. https://www.cdc.gov/nchs/fastats/asthma.htm. Accessed 20 Jan 2022

CDC (2021c) Childhood obesity facts. Centers for disease control and prevention. https://www.cdc.gov/obesity/data/childhood.html. Accessed 20 Jan 2022

CDC (2021d) Deaths by race and Hispanic origin, ages 0–18 years. Centers for Disease Control and Prevention. https://data.cdc.gov/nchs/deaths-by-race-and-hispanic-origin-ages-0-18-years/32c3-mvuz. Accessed 20 Jan 2022

Chu L, Elliott M, Stein E et al (2021) Identifying and managing suicidality in myalgic encephalomyelitis/chronic fatigue syndrome. Healthcare (Basel). 2021 Jun; 9(6):629. https://doi.org/10.3390/healthcare9060629

Davis J (2021) 560 Healthcare providers fell victim to ransomware attacks in 2020. health it security. https://healthitsecurity.com/news/560-healthcare-providers-fell-victim-to-ransomware-attacks-in-2020. Accessed 20 Jan 2022

Dennis A, Wamil M, Alberts J On behalf of COVERSCAN study investigators et al (2021) Multiorgan impairment in low-risk individuals with post-COVID-19 syndrome: a prospective, community-based study. BMJ Open 11:e048391. https://doi.org/10.1136/bmjopen-2020-048391

Disability Rights Texas (2021a) Federal judge rules governor order banning mask mandates violates federal law. Disability Rights Texas. November 10, 2021. https://www.disabilityrightstx.org/en/press_release/mask-mandate-ban-violates-federal-law/. Accessed 20 Jan 2022

Disability Rights Texas (2021b) First federal lawsuit filed against Texas governor on mask mandate ban says it violates ADA, section 504. Disability Rights Texas. August 17, 2021. https://www.disabilityrightstx.org/en/press_release/federal-lawsuit-texas-mask-mandate-ban/. Accessed 20 Jan 2022

Douaud G, Lee S, Alfaro-Almagro F et al (2021) Brain imaging before and after COVID-19 in UK Biobank. MedRxiv. https://doi.org/10.1101/2021.06.11.21258690

Guise J, McVittie C, McKinlay A (2010) A discourse analytic study of ME/CFS (Chronic Fatigue Syndrome) sufferers' experiences of interactions with doctors. J Hea Psy. https://doi.org/10.1177/1359105309350515

Israel Ministry of Health (2021) Results of the long-COVID survey among children in Israel. Israel ministry of health. https://www.gov.il/en/departments/news/13092021-01. Accessed 20 Jan 2022

Johnson BD, Vanatta N, Coon C (2021) Threatcasting (synthesis lectures on threatcasting). Morgan & Claypool. San Rafael

Kang C (2021) Facebook whistle-blower urges lawmakers to regulate the company. New York times. https://www.nytimes.com/2021/10/05/technology/facebook-whistle-blower-hearing.html. Accessed 20 Jan 2022

Koma W, Cubanski J, Neuman T (2021) Medicare and telehealth: coverage and use during the COVID-19 pandemic and options for the future. Kaiser Family Foundation. https://www.kff.org/medicare/issue-brief/medicare-and-telehealth-coverage-and-use-during-the-covid-19-pandemic-and-options-for-the-future/. Accessed 20 Jan 2022

Lowrey A (2021) The time tax. The Atlantic. https://www.theatlantic.com/politics/archive/2021/07/how-government-learned-waste-your-time-tax/619568/. Accessed 20 Jan 2022

Madgavkar A, White O, Krishnan M et al (2020) COVID-19 and gender equality: Countering the regressive effects. McKinsey Global Institute. https://www.mckinsey.com/featured-insights/future-of-work/covid-19-and-gender-equality-countering-the-regressive-effects. Accessed 20 Jan 2022

Maldonado S (2021) Some nyc workers battling 'long COVID' find chances for accommodations remote. The City NYC. https://www.thecity.nyc/2021/9/29/22701341/nyc-long-covid-workers-seek-remote-accomodations. Accessed 20 Jan 2022

McCormick D, Richardson L, Young P et al (2021) Deaths in children and adolescents associated with COVID-19 and mis-c in the United States. Pediatrics. https://doi.org/10.1542/peds.2021-052273

Moyer M (2019) People drawn to conspiracy theories share a cluster of psychological features. Scientific American. https://www.scientificamerican.com/article/people-drawn-to-conspiracy-theories-share-a-cluster-of-psychological-features/. Accessed 20 Jan 2022

Mundell E, Preidt R (2021) Many Show long-term organ damage after COVID. WebMD. https://www.webmd.com/lung/news/20210401/many-show-long-term-organ-damage-after-covid. Accessed 20 Jan 2022

Nakashima E, Shaban H, Lerman R (2021) The Biden administration seeks to rally allies and the private sector against the ransomware threat. Washington Post. https://www.washingtonpost.com/business/2021/06/04/white-house-fbi-ransomware-attacks/. Accessed 20 Jan 2022

Ollove M (2021) Long COVID renews push to expand palliative care. Pew Research Center. https://www.pewtrusts.org/en/research-and-analysis/blogs/stateline/2021/04/20/long-haul-covid-renews-push-to-expand-palliative-care. Accessed 20 Jan 2022

Price C, Vardavas R (2020) COVID-19 could become a widespread preexisting condition in a post-aca world. RAND Corporation. https://www.rand.org/blog/2020/11/covid-19-could-become-a-widespread-pre-existing-condition.html. Accessed 20 Jan 2022

SSA (2022) Social Security: What's New in 2022? Social Security Administration. https://www.ssa.gov/redbook/newfor2022.htm. Accessed 20 Sept 2022

Stoller K (2021) Never want to go back to the office? here's where you should work. Forbes. https://www.forbes.com/sites/kristinstoller/2021/01/31/never-want-to-go-back-to-the-office-heres-where-you-should-work/?sh=21a397a96712. Accessed 20 Jan 2022

Stone W (2022) CDC's new COVID metrics can leave individuals struggling to understand their risk. National Public Radio. https://www.npr.org/sections/health-shots/2022/03/10/1085797307/cdcs-new-COVID-metrics-can-leave-individuals-struggling-to-understand-their-risk. Accessed 20 Sept 2022

Turkewitz J, Linderman J (2012) The disability trap. New York Times. https://www.nytimes.com/2012/10/21/sunday-review/the-trap-of-supplemental-security-income.html. Accessed 20 Jan 2022

US Congress (2021) Text - S.2065 - 117th Congress (2021–2022) Supplemental security income restoration act of 2021. (2021, June 15). http://www.congress.gov/. Accessed 20 Jan 2022

Vogel S (2021) Prepare for a tsunami of long-COVID disability claims. HR Brew. https://www.morningbrew.com/hr/stories/2021/10/20/prepare-for-a-tsunami-of-long-COVID-disability-claims?utm_campaign=hrb&utm_medium=newsletter&utm_source=morning_brew. Accessed 20 Jan 2022

West D (2017) How to combat fake news and disinformation. Brookings Institute. https://www.brookings.edu/research/how-to-combat-fake-news-and-disinformation/. Accessed 20 Jan 2022

Wheeler L (2020) COVID unknowns leave survivors fearing life insurance rejection. Bloomberg. https://www.bloomberg.com/news/articles/2020-12-02/covid-unknowns-leave-survivors-fearing-life-insurance-rejection. Accessed 20 Jan 2022

Young R, McMahon S (2020) 'They're not actually getting better,' says founder of COVID-19 long-haulers support group. WBUR. https://www.wbur.org/hereandnow/2020/09/10/COVID-19-survivor-corps. Accessed 20 Jan 2022

Where Do We Go from Here?

6

The COVID-19 pandemic was a mass disabling event, and the emerging public health crisis of Long COVID has few modern analogs that can truly predict its full societal impact. A substantial policy response is needed to address this crisis as individually-focused solutions cannot sustainably or effectively combat the scope of the problem. When the Threatcasting pilot project was run in the fall of 2021, much of the information about Long COVID that was needed to make decisions about the disease was still emerging—stalling progress on the issue.

Since then, more substantial information about the biological underpinnings and social impact of Long COVID has emerged. However, the uptake of this information by the policy makers responsible for initiating an appropriate response is still incomplete. More education and awareness on the long-term impacts of COVID-19 and how this issue will intersect with other policy concerns are needed across all levels of government. Additionally, research on Long COVID that is focused on biomarkers, diagnostics, and treatment needs to be funded and accelerated.

Existing knowledge on illnesses that indicate a large degree of overlap with Long COVID, such as ME/CFS, can and should be used to inform this research effort and allow Long COVID research to simultaneously benefit the millions of people living with neglected post-infectious illness. Until this research can be translated into clinical outcomes, economic stopgap and safety net policies need to be expanded to ensure that people suddenly disabled by Long COVID can survive long enough to benefit from this research.

© The Author(s), under exclusive license to Springer Nature Switzerland AG 2024   101
M. Smallwood, *The Future of Long COVID*, Synthesis Lectures on Threatcasting,
https://doi.org/10.1007/978-3-031-40474-0_6

6.1   Healthcare

As a new disease and emerging public health crisis, research on the causes and potential treatments for Long COVID is nascent and will underlie much of the healthcare given to Long COVID patients moving forward. However, there is a substantial need for biomedical research on Long COVID to be funded and conducted—with clinical trials of potential treatments being a particularly urgent need that many members of the Long COVID community are more than willing to accept the risks of. In addition to basic biomedical research on Long COVID, targeted research needs to be conducted on topics and populations that require special consideration. These topics include the following:

1. The long-term impacts of COVID-19 and Long COVID on children;
2. The unique needs and barriers to care faced by Long COVID patients from communities of color, rural populations, and other marginalized groups;
3. Experiences with Long COVID outside of a Western context; and
4. The neurological and psychiatric impacts of Long COVID.

Any research into Long COVID should make a concerted effort to prioritize patient voices and expertise through collaboration with the highly active long-hauler research community, as well as chronic illness communities that existed before the pandemic and have informed much of the current Long COVID movement. The Patient-Centered Outcomes Research Institute (PCORI) was created specifically to fund this type of collaboration between medical research and patient advocates. However, broader Long COVID research funded by the NIH would also benefit from patient inclusion and collaboration.

Healthcare agencies such as the CDC and HHS, hospital systems, and professional organizations within the medical community should take steps to improve provider and public knowledge about Long COVID and other forms of complex chronic illness. Because COVID-19 can attack nearly every organ and bodily system in unpredictable ways, the medical aftereffects of the pandemic are likely to manifest in a wide range of outpatient specialties and settings. Despite this, many healthcare practitioners have limited knowledge about providing the appropriate treatment for patients with complex chronic illness. More effort should be made to disseminate knowledge collected by the Long COVID and ME/CFS research communities to practitioners in other specialties through continuing education programs.

Primary care and pediatric providers need to be educated on Long COVID since their offices are the first stop for Long COVID patients in the healthcare system. A lack of knowledge about Long COVID in a primary care setting can derail Long COVID patients' efforts to receive a diagnosis and appropriate care. Primary care referrals are often a necessary step for Long COVID patients to access specialized services through a post-COVID clinic, and misdiagnosis or the dismissal of Long COVID symptoms as anxiety or psychosomatic illness can prohibit these patients from receiving appropriate care.

After being assessed at a post-COVID clinic, a patient's care plan will often involve management through a primary care provider—which a provider who is educated on Long COVID will be better equipped to manage. Incorporating screenings for common post-COVID medical issues into routine medical practice in settings such as primary care can help catch these health issues early on and direct patients toward managing these conditions appropriately. Such a practice can also help maintain awareness of the medical aftereffects of COVID-19 among both practitioners and the general public.

6.2   Economic Support

Addressing the economic issues associated with Long COVID involves two main populations—long-haulers who are unable to work, and long-haulers who are able to work with accommodations. Each of these two broad coalitions has unique challenges that fall into different policy areas. Long-haulers who are no longer able to work must contend with the federal disability system (SSI)—a long-underfunded system that is at risk of being overwhelmed by a deluge of long-hauler disability claims. One of the major issues currently faced by long-haulers is the denial of disability claims and benefits. Although the Biden administration has stated that Long COVID will be considered a disability under the ADA, there are a considerable number of obstacles between this declaration and addressing the myriad barriers that are preventing many long-haulers from actually receiving these benefits. Insurance companies face little consequence for denying benefits to long COVID patients or forcing them to endure long legal and bureaucratic battles to receive assistance. Greater effort needs to be put toward resolving this current diagnostic and legal quagmire that is forcing long-haulers into economic desperation.

Establishing and expanding medium-term financial assistance options for long-haulers needs to be a policy priority. Currently, Long COVID patients who are working their way through the slow systems in place for long-term disability support must rely on a network of short-term safety net programs such as the Family and Medical Leave Act (FMLA). For long-haulers infected during the first wave of the pandemic, these time-limited safety net programs are running out, despite the disabilities experienced by these patients having no end in sight. Long COVID defies the conceptions of disability that underlie the existing disability support system, as an unpredictable, long-term, severe illness with a rapid acute onset. As a result, neither the short-term nor long-term disability support systems are equipped to handle it.

For long-haulers who have been able to maintain their employment, workplace accommodations and flexibility are essential for allowing them to sustainably balance their health and employment. The rapid adoption of technologies allowing remote work across entire sectors of the workforce during the pandemic has proved that these sorts of accommodations are not only possible, but that they are beneficial to employees with a wide range of needs—including those with disabilities, young children, or caregiving responsibilities.

Maintaining and normalizing the use of remote work and work flexibility across sectors that have already proven capable of using these options will be the most effective way to allow long-haulers to remain employed, and for employers to maintain their current workforce. An unaddressed, but important issue within this space is the lack of solutions for long-haulers whose jobs require physical, in-person work. This is likely to be a major problem moving forward, especially for in-person labor sectors with high rates of COVID exposure, and low-income and rural Americans who do not have access to jobs that allow remote work as an option.

6.3   Addressing the Needs of Children

The mass infection of children by the Omicron variants and lack of mitigations within schools indicates that a majority of American children have been infected with COVID-19—and therefore, are at risk of developing Long COVID and other physical or psychiatric conditions. Not all children infected by the virus will experience these ill effects, but pediatricians, teachers, school administrators, and other professionals charged with the well-being of children need to anticipate that disabilities and chronic conditions will be more common in the current cohort of school-aged children than in previous generations.

Without appropriate diagnosis and support, these disabilities—particularly those that are cognitive or neuropsychiatric—place children at risk of falling behind in school and failing to successfully transition to college or the workforce. These children are likely to need educational supports such as Individualized Education Programs (IEPs). Currently, IEP resources are available for children with ME/CFS, dyslexia, ADHD, and other learning disabilities who have similar needs as children with Long COVID (Duarte 2018), and this pre-existing knowledge should be used to inform the development of Long COVID-specific IEPs. Greater awareness and education on Long COVID also needs to be disseminated to pediatricians, educators, school administrators, and other professionals who will be interacting with children who are trying to succeed in the face of post-COVID disability.

The impact of COVID-19 and Long COVID on pediatric populations, particularly regarding neurodevelopmental effects, is a research gap that needs to be addressed with longitudinal studies on this topic. The development of screening tools for common post-COVID health issues in children, to be used in settings such as pediatric primary care or school health screenings, could help address the barriers to diagnosis and support faced by many children experiencing post-COVID issues. However, such a program would require greater investment in education—an investment that has been long deprioritized in many states—and may be politically fraught due to recent intense politicization of schools and education.

6.4   Politics and the Information Ecosystem

Political polarization, congressional gridlock, online misinformation, and a cultural push towards COVID normalization are among the most challenging of the issues raised in this Threatcasting workshop that impact the lives and futures of the millions of people living with Long COVID. Although many of the groups raised these issues in the threat scenarios, there were few proposed solutions to these problems that did not involve the removal of long-standing institutional barriers and frightening political trends that show few signs of reversing or slowing down. In many cases, these structural political issues are the main barriers preventing obvious policies that would strengthen the social safety net and aid in pandemic recovery from being passed into law.

Addressing political dysfunction on both the state and federal level is an urgent, but difficult task that requires long-term action and will likely face steep political opposition. For patients, healthcare providers, and policymakers who are trying to address issues surrounding Long COVID, it may be wisest to consider where coordinated political action may be most effective and what sorts of policy priorities are the most feasible to achieve in the short-term, versus what may only be politically viable through long-term change. However, it is essential that we continue to conceptualize Long COVID as a long-term issue facing our world, with the effects of the COVID-19 pandemic as a mass-disabling event continuing to manifest decades from our current moment. Any robust policy action on addressing Long COVID needs to look beyond the short-term political cycles that drive much of our current policy-making, and take a long-term approach to strengthening the healthcare, research, infrastructure and social systems that will allow us to handle this ongoing crisis. This approach will not only help mitigate the worst long-term effects of COVID-19. It is this type of thinking and policy making that is needed to address the multitude of complex problems facing our increasingly chaotic and interconnected world.

Reference

Duarte, L (2018) back to school part 2: IEPS for students with ME/CFS in public schools [Video File]. https://www.youtube.com/watch?v=zlcstzelsri. Accessed 20 Jan 2022

Conclusion

The COVID-19 pandemic has proven to be the deadliest and most disruptive public health crisis in recent history, rivaled only by the 1918 influenza pandemic. This novel virus has infected hundreds of millions of people around the world and imposed long-term risks to the future health, well-being, and prosperity of many of them. The long-term threats that Long COVID poses to both individuals and society arise from the medical impacts of the illness itself, and public support systems that are underfunded and ill-equipped to handle widespread, population-level disability. As with many other aspects of the COVID-19 pandemic, the challenges posed to systems and institutions by Long COVID are not new, but are instead exacerbations of long-standing systemic issues in American society. In many cases, the programs and policies meant to address the needs of people with complex disabilities such as Long COVID exist in a technical sense, but are too underfunded, underutilized, or hindered by political fighting to provide solutions to the people they are meant to serve.

Many of the factors that exacerbated the severity of the COVID-19 pandemic in the US are tied to cultural ableism that devalues disabled lives while conceptualizing disability as a niche issue affecting a small minority of the population whose needs have no bearing on the rest of the "normal" population. The COVID-19 pandemic exposed not only the inaccuracy of this idea but also the risks that widespread ignorance, neglect, and siloing of disability issues pose to public health. In a short period of time, the medical aftereffects of COVID-19 transformed disability from a niche issue to one affecting—and uniting—millions of people from all walks of life. Much of the work that has been done to define and raise awareness around Long COVID has been done by the sickest and most severely affected among us—newly disabled long-haulers working in conjunction with patients

M. Smallwood, *The Future of Long COVID*, Synthesis Lectures on Threatcasting, https://doi.org/10.1007/978-3-031-40474-0_7

suffering from ME/CFS and other complex chronic illnesses who have been neglected by the medical system for decades.

As the COVID-19 pandemic persists and more information surfaces about the long-term effects of this virus, our society stands at an inflection point. How we move forward in addressing the needs of the millions of people who have become newly disabled by COVID-19 will fundamentally shift how our society thinks about, cares for, and includes individuals with disabilities. Or else, we risk repeating past injustices and mistakes on a mass scale. A policy response on multiple levels—federal and local, legislative and regulatory, public and private—is needed to address and mitigate the threats that population-level disability caused by Long COVID poses to our society.

A wealth of information on Long COVID and the needs of COVID survivors has already been collected and organized by the patient-led research groups and social networks that first identified the condition. Collaboration and sustained relationships between long-hauler networks and policymakers are vital to ensuring that policy surrounding Long COVID meets the needs of the people it is meant to help.

A monumental task stands before us—one that only grows greater by the day as the COVID-19 pandemic drags on. Only by recognizing the true threat posed by the long-term effects of the virus and acting in solidarity with those most affected can we begin to move forward and break the cycles that created this situation.